Breathing in America: Diseases, Progress, and Hope

Breathing in America: Diseases, Progress, and Hope

Edited by Dean E. Schraufnagel, MD

Managing Editor
Brian Kell, MA

Art Director
Dorcas Gelabert, MFA

Illustration
Wendolyn B. Hill, MFA, CMI

Assistant Editor
Keely Savoie, MA

Editorial Assistant
Blythe Pack, MSW

Published by the American Thoracic Society, which gratefully acknowledges support and technical review from the National Heart, Lung, and Blood Institute, National Institutes of Health.

ISBN: 978-0-615-38058-2

Typesetter: MPS Limited, A Macmillan Company
Project manager: Manoj Kumar
Cover design: Dorcas Gelabert

Table of Contents

Editorial Contributors

Timothy R. Aksamit, MD
Consultant, Mayo Clinic

Donna J. Appell, RN
President and Founder
Hermansky-Pudlak Syndrome Network Inc.

Eric Bonura, MD
Fellow, Division of Pulmonary and Critical
    Care Medicine
New York University School of Medicine

Alice M. Boylan, MD
Associate Professor of Medicine
Director, Medical Acute and Critical Care
Medical University of South Carolina
Division of Pulmonary and Critical Care

V. Courtney Broaddus, MD
Professor of Medicine
Chief, Division of Pulmonary and
    Critical Care Medicine
San Francisco General Hospital
Associate Director
Lung Biology Center
University of California at San Francisco

David W. Brown, MScPH, MSc
Centers for Disease Control and Prevention

William W. Busse, MD
George R. and Elaine Love Professor
Chair, Department of Medicine
University of Wisconsin School of Medicine
    and Public Health

John W. Christman, MD
Professor of Medicine and Pharmacology
Section of Pulmonary, Critical Care,
    Sleep, and Allergy
University of Illinois at Chicago

Stephen C. Crane, PhD, MPH
Executive Director
American Thoracic Society

Janet B. Croft, PhD
Senior Epidemiologist
National Center for Chronic Disease
    Prevention and Health Promotion
Centers for Disease Control and Prevention

J. Randall Curtis, MD, MPH
Professor of Medicine
University of Washington
Harborview Medical Center

Charles L. Daley, MD
Head, Division of Mycobacterial and
    Respiratory Infections
National Jewish Health
Professor of Medicine
University of Colorado Denver

Fran DuMelle, MS
Senior Director, International Programs
    and Activities
American Thoracic Society

Gary Ewart, MHS
Senior Director of Government Relations
American Thoracic Society

Karen A. Fagan, MD
Associate Professor of Medicine
Chief, Division of Pulmonary Sciences and
    Critical Care Medicine
University of South Alabama

Reda E. Girgis, MB BCh
Associate Professor of Medicine
Co-Director, Pulmonary Hypertension Program
Associate Medical Director, Lung
    Transplantation
Johns Hopkins University

Chadi A. Hage, MD
Assistant Professor of Medicine
Pulmonary-Critical Care Medicine and
    Infectious Diseases
Indiana University School of Medicine
Roudebush VA Medical Center

Anna R. Hemnes, MD
Assistant Professor of Medicine
Assistant Director
Pulmonary Vascular Center
Division of Allergy, Pulmonary and Critical
    Care Medicine
Vanderbilt University School of Medicine

Nicholas S. Hill, MD
Professor of Medicine
Tufts University School of Medicine
Chief, Division of Pulmonary, Critical Care
    and Sleep Medicine
Tufts Medical Center

Leonard D. Hudson, MD
Professor of Medicine
Division of Pulmonary and Critical Care
    Medicine
University of Washington

Michael C. Iannuzzi, MD, MBA
Professor and Chair
Department of Medicine
SUNY Upstate Medical University

David Ingbar, MD
Professor of Medicine, Physiology & Pediatrics
Director of Pulmonary, Allergy and
    Critical Care Division
University of Minnesota

Manu Jain, MD, MS
Associate Professor of Medicine and Pediatrics
Director of Adult Cystic Fibrosis Program
Northwestern University Feinberg School of
    Medicine

Min J. Joo, MD, MPH
Assistant Professor of Medicine
Section of Pulmonary, Critical Care Sleep,
    and Allergy
University of Illinois at Chicago

Brian Kell, MA
Senior Director of Communications
    and Marketing
American Thoracic Society

James P. Kiley, PhD
Director of the Division of Lung Diseases
National Heart, Lung, and Blood Institute

Landon S. King, MD
David Marine Professorship in Medicine
Director, Pulmonary and Critical
    Care Medicine
Johns Hopkins School of Medicine

Alan R. Leff, MD
Professor of Medicine
University of Chicago

Yong Liu, MPH
Biostatistician, Division of Adult and
    Community Health
National Center for Chronic Disease
    Prevention and Health Promotion
Centers for Disease Control and Prevention

Robert Loddenkemper, MD
Professor of Medicine,
Charité Universitätsmedizin Berlin
Former Medical Director of
HELIOS Klinikum Emil von Behring
and Chief of Department of Pneumology II at
Lungenklinik Heckeshorn (Berlin)

Lisa A. Maier, MD, MSPH
Head, Division of Occupational &
    Environmental Health Sciences
National Jewish Health
Associate Professor of Medicine
University of Colorado Denver

David M. Mannino, MD
Associate Professor of Medicine
Division of Pulmonary, Critical Care,
    and Sleep Medicine
Director of the Pulmonary Epidemiology
    Research Laboratory
University of Kentucky

Susanna A. McColley, MD
Associate Professor of Pediatrics
Northwestern University Feinberg School
    of Medicine
Head, Division of Pulmonary Medicine
Director, Cystic Fibrosis Center

Francis X. McCormack, MD
Taylor Professor and Division Director
Pulmonary, Critical Care & Sleep Medicine
University of Cincinnati

Alfred Munzer, MD
Director of Pulmonary Medicine
Washington Adventist Hospital

John H. Newman, MD
Elsa S. Hanigan Professor of
    Pulmonary Medicine
Division of Allergy, Pulmonary and
    Critical Care Medicine
Vanderbilt University School of Medicine

Amy L. Olson, MD, MSPH
Assistant Professor
Interstitial Lung Disease Program
National Jewish Health

Marc Peters-Golden, MD
Professor of Internal Medicine
Director, Fellowship Program in Pulmonary
    and Critical Care Medicine
University of Michigan Health System

Bharati Prasad, MD
Assistant Professor
University of Illinois Medical Center
    at Chicago

J. Usha Raj, MD
Professor and Head
Department of Pediatrics
University of Illinois at Chicago

William N. Rom, MD, MPH
Sol and Judith Bergstein Professor of Medicine
Director, Division of Pulmonary and
    Critical Care Medicine
New York University School of Medicine

Jesse Roman, MD
Professor and Chairman of Medicine
University of Louisville Health Sciences Center

Keely Savoie, MA
Science Writer and Senior Media Liaison
American Thoracic Society

Dean E. Schraufnagel, MD
Professor of Medicine and Pathology
Section of Pulmonary, Critical Care,
    Sleep and Allergy
University of Illinois at Chicago

David A. Schwartz, MD
Director, Center for Genetics and Therapeutics
Provost, National Jewish Health

Marvin I. Schwarz, MD
Professor of Medicine
Co-Head, Division of Pulmonary Sciences
    and Critical Care Medicine
University of Colorado Health Sciences Center

Lynn T. Tanoue, MD
Professor of Medicine
Pulmonary and Critical Care Medicine
Yale University School of Medicine

Gerard Turino, MD
Founding Director
James P. Mara Center for Lung Disease
St. Luke's-Roosevelt Hospital Center
John H. Keating Sr. Professor of Medicine
    (Emeritus)
Columbia University College of Physicians
    & Surgeons

Adam Wanner, MD
Joseph Weintraub Professor of Medicine
University of Miami Miller School of Medicine

Ewald R. Weibel, MD, DSc (hon)
Professor Emeritus of Anatomy
Institute of Anatomy
University of Berne

Gail G. Weinmann, MD
Deputy Director of the Division of
    Lung Diseases
National Heart, Lung, and Blood Institute

Jo Rae Wright, PhD
Professor, Department of Cell Biology,
    Pediatrics and Medicine
Vice Provost & Dean of the Graduate School
Duke University School of Medicine

Zhi-Jie Zheng, MD, MPH, PhD
Senior Medical Epidemiologist and
Program Director, Research Translation
Division for the Application of Research
    Discoveries
National Heart, Lung, and Blood Institute

Foreword

Respiratory issues affect millions of Americans, robbing them of their health, happiness, and even of life itself. Asthma, COPD, lung cancer, and sleep apnea are just a few of the important respiratory conditions that pose major threats to our citizens. Just as importantly, airborne threats such as influenza, air pollution, and bioterrorism can spread rapidly through the air, affecting enormous numbers of people in a very short period of time. Moreover, tobacco smoke kills more Americans in one year than all the wars our nation fought during the last century.

Congress has recognized the importance of respiratory health and has embarked on programs to make a difference. From 1998–2003, Congress doubled the budget of the National Institutes of Health. We have strengthened the Centers for Disease Control and Prevention, granted the Food and Drug Administration the ability to regulate tobacco, improved pollution control through the Environmental Protection Agency, and funded tuberculosis programs throughout the world to control tuberculosis at home.

The money invested in research has been money well spent. Americans are living longer and healthier and, for the most part, breathing easier. Some previously untreatable diseases, such as respiratory distress of the newborn—once a leading cause of infant mortality—now have treatments; others have cures within their grasp.

Research is essential for the United States to remain a world leader in the development of health advances. The benefits of research extend beyond healthy citizens. Research improves our nation's productivity, increases employment, and improves the financial well-being of our citizens. More progress must be made, both in understanding disease processes in order to develop cures and in bringing these advances to everyone.

I congratulate the American Thoracic Society on this book, which highlights many of the advances that recent research has brought about and demonstrates the value of working together to improve the lung health of Americans.

Mike Crapo
United State Senator, Idaho

Preface

Breathing in America: Diseases, Progress, and Hope briefly describes respiratory diseases and the progress that is being made in the quest to find their cures. It describes who is vulnerable to developing these diseases, what it is like to have them, and their burden on society. It tells about prevention, treatment, and ways to stay healthy. And, most importantly, it explains where we are in understanding the disease processes, how close research is to developing new tests and treatments, and what still needs to be done.

Many factors went into developing this book. Nearly a decade ago, the European Respiratory Society sought to identify variations in lung diseases across different European nations. In 2003, it published the *European Lung White Book,* a report that helped to increase awareness of the high toll of lung diseases. The Forum for International Respiratory Societies, which is composed of organizations including the American Thoracic Society, the European Respiratory Society, the Asociación Latinoamericana del Tórax, the American College of Chest Physicians, the Asian Pacific Society of Respirology, the International Union Against Tuberculosis and Lung Disease, and the Pan African Thoracic Society, determined that a similar report should be completed for each region of the world. The American Thoracic Society agreed to undertake this project for the United States.

The American Thoracic Society frequently receives inquiries from the media, patients, and the public at large regarding specific lung diseases and scientific advances in respiratory research. To address these inquiries, staff members thought that a short review of respiratory diseases would be helpful. There have long been advocates within the American Thoracic Society for a publication that covered the topics now found in *Breathing in America: Diseases, Progress, and Hope.* The American Thoracic Society's Research Advocacy Committee, for example, believes that increased awareness of respiratory disease will expand support for respiratory research, which—by just about any measure—is underfunded when considering the number of lives affected. The committee produced a document that outlined the research that is needed and the areas where that research could make a major impact. The American Thoracic Society's Public Advisory Roundtable consists of patient advocacy groups for various respiratory and critical illnesses. This group strongly supports research, which they see as the best hope for improving the lives of people with respiratory diseases. Patient advocates remind us that the burden of lung diseases extends far beyond the numbers of persons who suffer or die from a respiratory illness.

These factors came together to become the impetus behind this book. Then American Thoracic Society President Jo Rae Wright, PhD, and the American Thoracic Society staff applied for a grant from the National Heart, Lung, and Blood Institute to allow production to begin.

The book is part of the American Thoracic Society's 2010 Year of the Lung campaign, an inclusion that required a short timeline to publication. The contributors, reviewers, and advisors carried out the needed tasks with amazing commitment, thoroughness, and promptness. None of it would have been possible without the great efforts of Brian Kell, the managing editor, who worked tirelessly to make this book happen.

Dean E. Schraufnagel, MD
Editor

Major Structures of the Lung

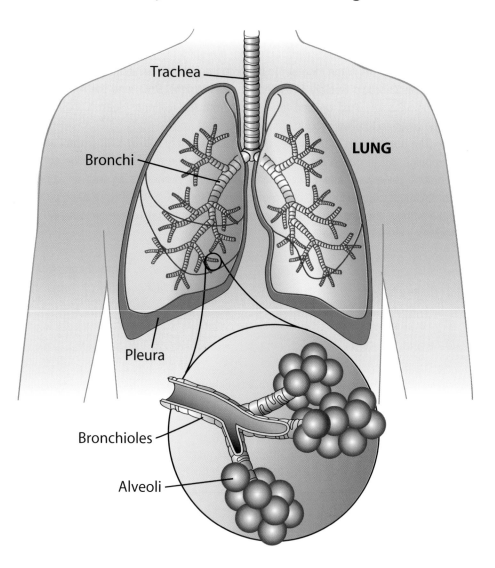

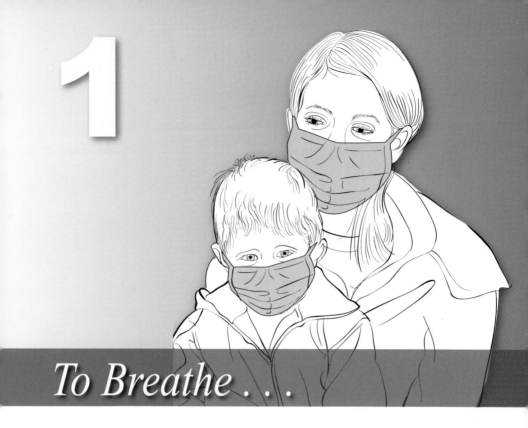

1

To Breathe . . .

To breathe is to live.

And yet people everywhere live with, and die from, breathing disorders. Those who suffer may be young or old. They may have a breathing problem from birth or develop it after years of working in certain environments. They may find that medical treatment can greatly relieve their symptoms or that little can be done to help them. They may live relatively normal lives or suffer major disability and an early death. They may wonder if a cure is around the corner or will not come in their lifetime.

The respiratory system suffers many onslaughts. Cigarette smoke, air pollution, and airborne infections are three major ones, but lack of awareness of the harm they do is an even greater danger. Together, respiratory diseases kill more than 400,000 Americans each year, making them the third-leading cause of death in the United States (1). For millions more, respiratory diseases significantly reduce quality of life. Being unable to breathe can be a terrifying experience, yet it is one that many face everyday.

Despite the commonplace and seriousness of respiratory conditions, they are often under-appreciated in discussions and decisions about public health. Perhaps this is because these conditions can take many forms. Some disorders, such as asthma, are common, affecting 19 million children and 16 million

Death rates for leading causes of death for all ages: United States, 1950–2005

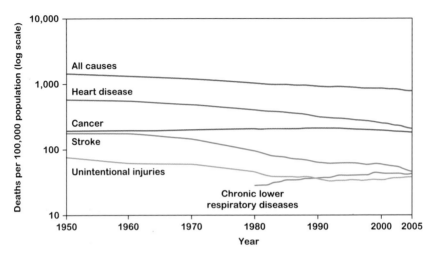

Of the six leading causes of death, only COPD (categorized as a chronic lower respiratory disease on the right) has become a more common cause over the past 30 years. National Center for Health Statistics. *Health, United States, 2008 With Chartbook.* Hyattsville, MD: 2009.

adults (2). Others, such as the Hermansky-Pudlak syndrome, are rare. Some, such as sarcoidosis, more commonly affect African Americans, while others, such as cystic fibrosis, more often affect Caucasians. Cystic fibrosis, one of the most common genetic disorders among Caucasians, manifests itself in early childhood. Lung fibrosis and lung cancer affect older adults. Still others, such as tuberculosis and sleep apnea, can strike at any age.

Many forms of lung disease disproportionately affect the socioeconomically disadvantaged, but all classes of people must breathe and no one, whether defined by age, gender, race, ethnicity, or socioeconomic level, is immune from respiratory problems and their potentially devastating impact.

Because populations share the same air, environmental exposures can affect large numbers of people, frequently at the same time. Infectious lung disease can be transmitted by humans, and environmental lung disease can be transmitted by human activity. Lung disease may result from as yet unknown factors in the air. And most lung diseases can occur without warning.

Lung cancer is the most common cause of cancer death in the United States and in the rest of the world. In the United States, more than 160,000 people died from lung cancer in 2009. That is more than from cancers of the breast, colon,

Age-adjusted cancer death rates, males by site, United States, 1930–2005

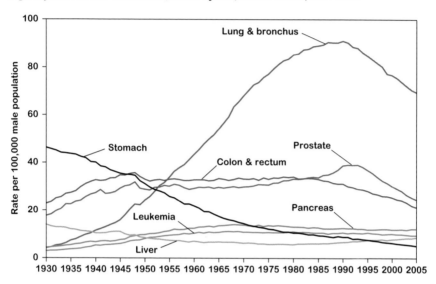

Age-adjusted cancer death rates, females by site, United States, 1930–2005

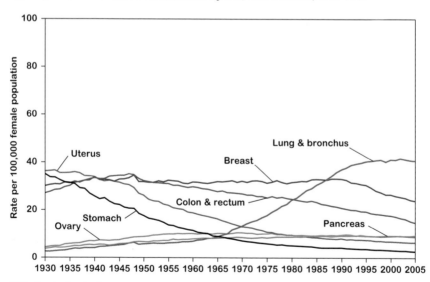

While the death rates from most cancers have stayed the same or decreased over the past 75 years, that for lung cancer have increased dramatically. Fortunately, among men, the death rate appears to have peaked in 1990. Among women, it also appears to have peaked, though more recently. American Cancer Society. *Cancer Facts and Figures 2009.* Atlanta: American Cancer Society; 2009.

pancreas, and prostate combined (3). More women die from lung cancer than from breast cancer.

Chronic obstructive pulmonary disease (COPD) affects 6.8 percent of adults (4) and is responsible for about 700,000 hospitalizations and 127,000 deaths annually in the United States (1,5). But more than half of people with COPD have not been diagnosed (6). Only heart disease, cancer, and stroke kill more people, but while deaths from those diseases are declining, the number of people dying from COPD is growing. By 2020, if recent mortality trends continue, COPD is expected to kill more Americans than stroke (7,8). Influenza and its sequelae pneumonia claim over 40,000 lives annually. Asthma, though usually not fatal, is also a growing problem. Among children, asthma cases more than doubled between 1980 and the mid-1990s; 6 percent of all American children now have asthma (9).

During the past two decades, sleep-disordered breathing has become recognized as a major health problem that may affect up to 10 percent of Americans. From 1990 to 2005, physician office visits for sleep apnea increased from 108,000 to 3.4 million in the United States, and yet most people with sleep apnea go undiagnosed and untreated (1).

Economic burden of lung disease

The economic cost of lung disease, both to individuals and to society, is vast. The U.S. Environmental Protection Agency estimated that in 1999, the average annual cost of treating a patient for asthma ranged from $761 to $889, depending on age (10). Asthma has other costs including missed time from school and work; school absences total about 12.8 million days per year. Costs are also borne by family members who need to miss work to obtain care for asthma, especially for children. The annual cost of asthma exceeds $19 billion per year in the United States (11,12). Researchers at a health economics firm estimated that the annual cost of providing COPD-related medical services was even higher, ranging in 2005 from $2,700 to $5,900 per person (13).

The National Heart, Lung, and Blood Institute estimated that in 2009, the annual cost of providing healthcare related to all respiratory conditions, excluding lung cancer, was $113 billion. The institute further estimated that the cost to American society, in terms of lost productivity as a result of disability and early death due to respiratory disease, amounted to an additional $67 billion (1).

A wonderful organ

The lung is a wonderful organ built of a complex tree of airways that are, in an average person, 44 miles long and serve to ventilate 300 to 500 million alveoli, or air sacs, with a total surface area nearly the size of a tennis court. This surface is covered by a dense meshwork of blood capillaries, whose total length is about 3,000 miles. About 85 percent of the alveolar surface is in contact with blood across a tissue barrier 50 times thinner than a sheet of onion skin paper, which allows a very efficient uptake of oxygen (14).

Breathing is regulated through a complex interaction between oxygen and carbon dioxide sensors located in the arteries and the brainstem, which respond to subtle changes in acidity. Sensors located in the lung and chest wall muscles respond to expansion and contraction, sending signals to the central respiratory controllers in the brainstem. The controllers help direct the respiratory muscles, triggering inspiration and expiration and regulating the depth of breathing. By expelling carbon dioxide, the lungs eliminate more acid waste in one hour than the kidneys do in an entire day.

The lung interacts with the environment

The lungs filter about 500 liters of air per hour or 12,000 liters per day. Inhaled air contains infectious and noxious particles and gases, against which the lungs must defend themselves. Mechanical factors, such as the structure of the nasal passageway and bronchi, and functional factors, such as cough, prevent invasion into the lung or expel invading elements. The thin layer of mucus, which traps particles and dissolves gases, is constantly propelled by hair-like structures, called *cilia*, up the bronchi to the trachea and mouth, where they are swallowed or expelled.

A variety of cells and lymphatic drainage also work to keep the lungs clear and relatively dry. The macrophage is a cell that originates in the bone marrow and migrates to the lung. It is capable of ingesting organisms and inert particles and of killing bacteria. After taking up the foreign material, macrophages may migrate up the bronchi and trachea to be swallowed or to the lymph nodes, where they initiate an inflammatory or immune response. This response may defend against infectious agents, but it can also provoke or be part of respiratory diseases themselves.

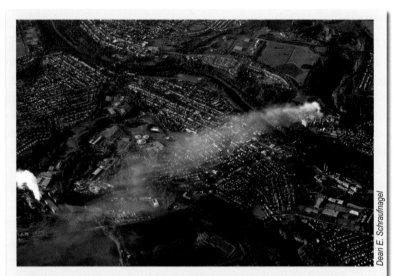

An aerial view of a smokestack shows how quickly and extensively airborne material spreads and why diseases such as influenza and tuberculosis can be so devastating. Airborne particles can be toxic in quantities as small as a few parts per billion.

Percentage of Americans who smoke

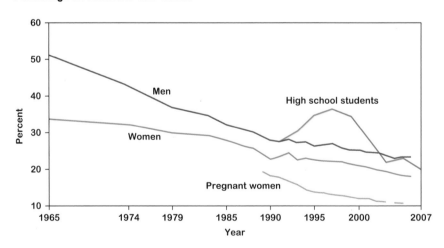

Most smokers start in their teenage years. The rise in adolescent smoking rates in the late 1990s may have been due to tobacco industry advertising that targeted youth. The subsequent decline is associated with increased prevention efforts by many states to curb advertising and offer counter-marketing messages. National Center for Health Statistics. *Health, United States, 2008 With Chartbook.* Hyattsville, MD: 2009.

To Breathe . . .

How lung disease happens

The complexity of the respiratory system does not lend itself to easy classification of its diseases, but one basic way to group them is by how they affect pulmonary function, or breathing, tests. Diseases that affect the flow of air are termed *obstructive lung diseases* and include asthma, emphysema, bronchitis, bronchiolitis, and bronchiectasis. The airflow obstruction is primarily in the passageways to the alveoli, where oxygen and carbon dioxide exchange takes place. Asthma is an inflammatory or allergic condition but is distinguished by its reversibility whereas the other conditions are not fully reversible. Bronchitis is an inflammation of the bronchi, and bronchiolitis is an inflammation of the bronchioles, the next segment of the airway that conducts air down to the alveoli. Emphysema is characterized by a loss of lung elasticity that occurs when the lungs are stretched at full inhalation. The loss of elasticity allows the lungs to overinflate; the excessive stretching breaks alveolar walls, which leads to decreased area for oxygen and carbon dioxide exchange.

Diseases that decrease the volume of the lung are called *restrictive lung diseases*. These diseases, such as pulmonary fibrosis, make breathing difficult because of increased lung stiffness and the work it takes to breathe.

Lung diseases may also be classified according to the disease-causing process, such as genetic, developmental, neoplastic (cancer), vascular, inflammatory, infectious, and toxic. Among the clearly defined genetic disorders of the lung are cystic fibrosis and alpha-1 antitrypsin deficiency (a form of emphysema). The most common developmental abnormality is the infant respiratory distress syndrome (or respiratory distress of the newborn). Later-life developmental abnormalities of the spine, such as scoliosis or kyphosis, can also adversely affect breathing.

Lung disease may also involve the blood vessels in disorders such as pulmonary embolism, which is associated with reduced blood flow and impairment in oxygen uptake. More rare inflammation of the blood vessels (vasculitis) also occurs. Diseases marked by inflammation of the airway include COPD, asthma, and bronchitis. Many diseases involve inflammation of the alveoli and the tissue next to them (interstitium). Sarcoidosis and fibrosis are chronic inflammatory diseases; if the inflammation does not resolve and allow the restoration of the normal structure, then scarring, or fibrosis, results. Pulmonary fibrosis can be a deadly form of such scarring.

Respiratory infections can be caused by viruses, bacteria, fungi, protozoa, and larger parasites. Respiratory infections range from mild, such as the common cold or acute bronchitis, to devastating, such as the pneumonia caused by *Pneumocystis*, which occurs in persons with the human immunodeficiency virus (HIV). Infectious agents may gain entry through the airway or the bloodstream. Overwhelming bloodstream infection is termed *sepsis*.

Because the lungs are in constant contact with the environment, they are especially susceptible to environmental toxins. Air pollution and toxic gases cause a variety of respiratory problems. Assaults on the lung can come from inhaling fumes or other noxious particles in the environment, such as tobacco smoke, or from material that gains access to the lung from the bloodstream (emboli). Exposure to high-oxygen concentrations can induce permanent lung injury, even when given as a life-saving medical treatment.

If lung disease advances rapidly, it can lead to acute respiratory failure. If lung disease progresses slowly, it can lead to chronic respiratory failure. Respiratory failure is defined by the lungs' inability to maintain a sufficient level of oxygen in the body or to clear carbon dioxide adequately. Respiratory failure can also result from weakness of respiratory muscles and from abnormalities of the chest wall and in the neural control of respiration. Impaired control of breathing in the central nervous system can cause sleep apnea, and delayed development of control of breathing in the brainstem has been invoked as a cause of sudden infant death syndrome.

The changing face of lung disease

At the beginning of the 20th century, infectious diseases were identified as the cause of enormous public health problems (15). Each year, tuberculosis claimed more than 2 of every 1,000 American lives in the United States (16). Scientists knew what tuberculosis looked like under the microscope, but there was no treatment. Today, scientists have deciphered the entire genome of *Mycobacterium tuberculosis* and are able to cure tuberculosis—but not in everyone.

Although infectious diseases were thought to be conquered through scientific advances, new microbial forms and altered human hosts (as seen with acquired immune deficiency syndrome [AIDS]) have led to their resurgence. In the early 20th century, influenza claimed 20 million lives around the globe. Today, the ill effects of influenza have been reduced by vaccines and medications—but

Major common lung diseases

Diseases of air movement and airways
Asthma
Bronchiectasis
Emphysema and chronic bronchitis (Chronic obstructive pulmonary disease, or COPD)
Bronchiolitis

Infectious lung diseases
Pneumonia (and lung abscess)
Pleural infections (empyema)
Fungal lung disease
Tuberculosis and other mycobacterial disease
Opportunistic lung infections in immunosuppressed persons

Pulmonary vascular diseases
Pulmonary embolism
Pulmonary hypertension
Congenital vascular anomalies

Congenital, genetic, and developmental lung diseases
Cystic fibrosis
Respiratory distress of the newborn
Alpha-1 antitrypsin deficiency
Congenital lung disease
Bronchopulmonary dysplasia
Congenital syndromes affecting the lungs

Lung cancers
Benign lung tumors
Lung carcinoma
Cancer metastatic to the lung

(*continued on next page*)

Environmental, exposure-related, and occupational lung diseases

Mineral dust pneumoconiosis (asbestosis, silicosis, coal workers' pneumoconiosis)

Hypersensitivity pneumonia (organic material exposure)

Drug-induced lung disease

Occupational asthma

Toxic exposure

Interstitial lung diseases

Cryptogenic organizing pneumonitis

Hypersensitivity pneumonitis

Idiopathic pulmonary fibrosis

Interstitial lung disease associated with autoimmune disease

Nonspecific interstitial pneumonitis

Pulmonary Langerhans histiocytosis

Respiratory bronchiolitis-interstitial lung disease

Sarcoidosis

Lymphangioleiomyomatosis

Sleep-related and neuromuscular breathing disorders

Obstructive sleep apnea

Central sleep apnea

Amyotrophic lateral sclerosis

Myasthenia gravis

Traumatic spinal cord disease

Diseases of the pleura and chest wall

Pleural effusion

Mesothelioma

Kyphoscoliosis

Traumatic chest injury

(continued on next page)

Respiratory failure
Acute and chronic respiratory failure
Acute respiratory distress syndrome
Sepsis
Shock
Multi-organ failure

Systemic disease affecting the respiratory system
Many diseases primarily affecting other organs
Autoimmune diseases

the threat of new strains with great potential to spread and cause harm still looms.

At the beginning of the 20th century, infant mortality was 13 times greater than today (17,18), and respiratory distress of the newborn was unrecognized. Today, surfactant replacement therapy has nearly eliminated this condition—but infants still die of respiratory failure.

At the beginning of the 20th century, there was no effective treatment for pneumonia. Today, there are scores of antibiotics that target bacterial infections—but pneumonia still kills, even within hospitals.

At the beginning of the 20th century, the world had not reconciled the benefits of the industrial revolution with the risks it imposed on its workers or, through its smokestacks that polluted the air, to all people. Today, there are effective worker protection laws and a national commitment to clean air. The reductions in atmospheric ozone, oxides of nitrogen, and particulate pollution have resulted in better quality of life and healthier lungs—but pollution still shortens lives.

Largely as a result of these and other medical advances and the public health movement, life expectancy has increased over the past century from 47 to 76 years—but there are hazards afoot.

Lung health cannot be taken for granted. At the beginning of the 20th century, tobacco smoking and lung cancer were rare. Today, multinational tobacco enterprises promote a habit that kills 440,000 Americans every year, as many lives lost as in all the wars fought by our country in the last hundred years (19).

Over the past century, the world's population has grown from two to six billion, placing an ever-increasing strain on our fragile biosphere. New infections have emerged, and the success of modern medicine has brought its own challenges. Although antibiotics have saved lives, they have also resulted in the emergence of highly resistant bacteria, which cause life-threatening infections and prolong hospital confinement.

Against the background of significant progress are formidable new challenges. Each chapter in this book describes a major respiratory disease: whom it affects; what it is like to have the disease; what is being learned about the disease; how it can be prevented, treated, and managed; and how research is making a difference. The purpose of the book is to describe these diseases and the progress made toward controlling them in the hope that someday they will be eliminated. The recognition of the gains made and the goals that may be within our grasp should stir the will and determination for all Americans to breathe, and live, better.

References

1. National Heart, Lung, and Blood Institute. Disease statistics. Available at: http://www.nhlbi. nih.gov/about/factbook/chapter4.htm. Accessed February 20, 2010.
2. Tang EA, Matusi E, Wiesch DG, Samet JM. Epidemiology of asthma and allergic diseases. In: Adkinson NF Jr, Bochner BS, Busse WW, Holgate ST, Lemanske RF Jr, Simons FER, eds. *Middleton's Allergy Principles & Practice.* Volume 2. 7th ed. Philadelphia, PA: Mosby Elsevier; 2009:715–767.
3. Jemal A, Siegel R, Ward E, Hao Y, Xu J, Thun MJ. Cancer statistics, 2009. *CA Cancer J Clin* 2009;59:225–249.
4. Centers for Disease Control and Prevention. National health and nutrition examination survey. Available at: http://www.cdc.gov/nchs/nhanes.htm. Accessed February 20, 2010.
5. Centers for Disease Control and Prevention (CDC). Deaths from chronic obstructive pulmonary disease—United States, 2000–2005. *MMWR Morb Mortal Wkly Rep* 2008;57:1229–1232.
6. Mannino DM, Braman S. The epidemiology and economics of chronic obstructive pulmonary disease. *Proc Am Thorac Soc* 2007;4:502–506.
7. Jemal A, Ward E, Hao Y, Thun M. Trends in the leading causes of death in the United States, 1970–2002. *JAMA* 2005;294:1255–1259.
8. Lopez AD, Shibuya K, Rao C, Mathers CD, Hansell AL, Held LS, Schmid V, Buist S. Chronic obstructive pulmonary disease: current burden and future projections. *Eur Respir J* 2006;27:397–412.
9. Centers for Disease Control and Prevention. The state of childhood asthma, United States, 1980–2005. Available at: http://cdc.gov/nchs/data/ad/ad381.pdf.
10. US Environmental Protection Agency. http://epa.gov/oppt/coi/pubs/IV_2.pdf.
11. American Lung Association. Lung disease data: 2008. Available at: http://www.lungusa.org/ assets/documents/publications/lung-disease-data/LDD_2008.pdf. Accessed February 20, 2010.
12. US Department of Health and Human Services. Action against asthma: a strategic plan for the Department of Health and Human Services. Available at: http://aspe.hhs.gov/sp/asthma. Accessed February 20, 2010.
13. Foster TS, Miller JD, Marton JP, Caloyeras JP, Russell MW, Menzin J. Assessment of the economic burden of COPD in the U.S.: a review and synthesis of the literature. *COPD* 2006;3:211–218.
14. Weibel ER. What makes a good lung? *Swiss Med Wkly* 2009;139:375–386.
15. Centers for Disease Control and Prevention (CDC). Control of infectious diseases. *MMWR Morb Mortal Wkly Rep* 1999;48:621–629.
16. Armstrong GL, Conn LA, Pinner RW. Trends in infectious disease mortality in the United States during the 20th century. *JAMA* 1999;281:61–66.
17. Centers for Disease Control and Prevention (CDC). Healthier mothers and babies. *MMWR Morb Mortal Wkly Rep* 1999;48:849–858.
18. Wegman ME. Infant mortality in the 20th century, dramatic but uneven progress. *J Nutr* 2001;131:401S–408S.
19. Centers for Disease Control and Prevention (CDC). State-specific smoking-attributable mortality and years of potential life lost—United States, 2000–2004. *MMWR Morb Mortal Wkly Rep* 2009;58:29–33.

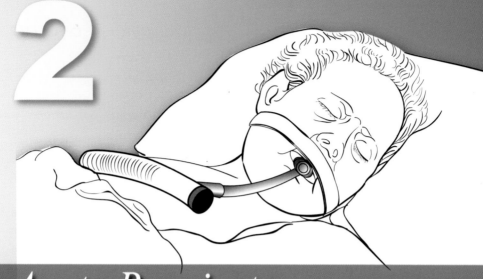

Acute Respiratory Distress Syndrome

Acute respiratory distress syndrome (ARDS) is a condition in which the lungs suffer severe widespread injury, interfering with their ability to take up oxygen. A low blood oxygen level and the inability to get oxygen to normal levels is the hallmark of ARDS. The term *acute* reflects the sudden onset—over minutes or hours—of an injury. Acute lung injury (ALI) is a more recently coined term that includes ARDS but also milder degrees of lung injury. ALI and ARDS always result from another severe underlying disease. The range of diseases causing ARDS is broad, and they may also damage organs other than the lungs, but the lung injury usually dominates the clinical picture (1).

The term *acute respiratory distress syndrome* was coined in 1967, with similar lung injury being recognized in both medical and surgical patients. About this same time, the condition was being widely recognized in severely wounded soldiers in the Vietnam War. The name was chosen in part to reflect similarities to the previously described infant respiratory distress syndrome in premature infants.

Although ARDS has undoubtedly always occurred, it has only been recognized in the modern medical era because more severely and acutely ill patients now survive long enough to develop lung injury as a complication of their underlying severe disease.

Whom does it affect?

Epidemiology, prevalence, economic burden, vulnerable populations

The occurrence of ARDS depends on several factors. Infectious diseases, which can result in ARDS, vary widely by geographic region. For example, malaria is the most frequent cause of ARDS in some parts of the world but does not exist in most of North America.

People at risk for ARDS are those with or at risk for the underlying diseases associated with the syndrome. The most common of these is sepsis, a severe infection that spreads throughout the body via the bloodstream. Victims of trauma and those who aspirate stomach contents into the lung are also at high risk for ARDS. A less common cause of direct injury is the inhalation of high concentrations of toxic gases, which can occur with severe smoke inhalation and in industrial accidents.

Age- and risk-specific incidence of mortality from acute lung injury

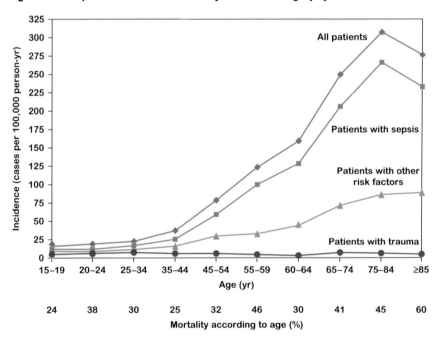

Sepsis is the most common condition leading to acute lung injury or acute respiratory distress syndrome. Mortality from both conditions is high and increases with age (2). Copyright © 2005 Massachusetts Medical Society. All rights reserved.

CASE STUDY

A 33-year-old woman developed back pain that worsened over several days. She took several medications, but the pain did not abate. After five days, she developed breathlessness and was hospitalized. The next day her blood pressure dropped and her kidneys failed. The following day, her breathing deteriorated and she required mechanical ventilation. Breathing became more difficult, and the high pressure required by the ventilator to get air into her lungs ruptured the lung alveoli, causing air to escape the lungs and be trapped inside the chest (pneumothorax). This was treated with a tube through the chest wall to allow the lungs to expand. She was deeply sedated to reduce the work required by her respiratory muscles. She developed pneumonia, and, after about three weeks on the ventilator, a new breathing tube was placed directly into the trachea (tracheostomy) in preparation for long-term mechanical ventilation. Fortunately, her kidney function returned, and she was able to clear the fluid in her lungs. Antibiotics treated the pneumonia. After four weeks in the hospital, the sedation was stopped, and after nine weeks, the tracheostomy tube was removed.

Comment

The woman, as most patients with ARDS who spend a prolonged time on a mechanical ventilator, did not recall much of the hospitalization. She remembered the rapidity with which she became ill and that several times she thought she was dying. For two years, she suffered from a form of post-traumatic stress disorder with flashbacks, but the flashbacks eventually stopped.

A recent study of Washington state's King County reflects the prevalence of acute lung injury and ARDS in North America. All patients with these conditions were identified in all hospitals of the county, a mixed urban and rural population that includes the city of Seattle. Seventy-nine people per 100,000 population per year developed ALI, and 59 of these met the criteria for the more severe form of ARDS. The death rate of ALI patients was 38.5 percent. Using the U.S. census and assuming the same frequency throughout the country, 190,600 people per year develop ALI, and 74,500 die of, or with, the disease in the United States. This makes ALI and ARDS diseases with major consequences to public health, causing about twice as many deaths per year as breast cancer or prostate cancer and several times more than HIV/AIDS (2). Yet, the general public is largely unaware of these common diseases.

What we are learning about the disease

Pathophysiology, causes: genetic, environment, microbes

The cause of the acute lung injury can be either direct, with the injurious agent reaching the lung through the airways or by trauma to the chest, or indirect, with the injurious agent arriving at the lungs through the bloodstream. The affected areas in ARDS are the alveoli (air sacs), where oxygen enters the blood and carbon dioxide leaves it (gas exchange). The thin wall between the blood and air is made up of the blood capillary and the alveolar wall (alveolar-capillary membrane). The alveolar-capillary membrane is extremely delicate, less than 0.5 micrometers in width at its thinnest segment where gas exchange takes place. (For comparison, an average human hair is about 100 micrometers in width.) In ARDS, both the capillary and alveolar cells are injured, whether the initiating process is direct or indirect. Injury to this membrane allows fluid to spill into the lung, thus hindering or preventing gas exchange.

The aspiration of stomach contents into the lung or the inhalation of toxic gases are examples of direct injury causing ARDS. Indirect lung injury, however, is a more common cause of ARDS and is usually associated with severe infections or severe trauma. Regardless of the initiating event, an inflammatory chain reaction is set off. Molecules released by infected or injured cells signal white cells from the blood to enter the affected area. The incoming white blood cells combine with resident cells to produce more chemicals (called *cytokines* and *chemokines*), which induce a variety of actions involved in the inflammatory process. Inflammation is usually beneficial, in that it promotes killing and containment of infectious agents and clearing of the debris created by the infection or injury. Occasionally, however, exuberant inflammation can spread beyond the originally damaged organ via the bloodstream to injure other organs and tissues at distant sites. This systemic process is called *sepsis* when the initiating insult is an infection, but a similar, if not identical, process can occur when the original insult is traumatic injury.

Sepsis or sepsis-like syndromes can cause injury and failure of many organs. When they affect the lungs, they most commonly cause ARDS. In patients with sepsis or sepsis-like syndromes, the lungs are often the first organ to be injured. They are often the most severely injured organ, and they frequently represent the only organ failure that is recognized clinically. This association may be because the lungs are the only organ to receive all the blood of the body. Although all the blood flows through the chambers of the heart, only a fraction of the blood supplies the heart tissues themselves. Thus the lungs receive the full brunt of the injurious cytokines and other molecules. The leakage of fluid through the alveolar-capillary membrane and flooding of alveoli interferes with oxygenation and causes shortness of breath and respiratory distress. The excess alveolar fluid mixes with the normal lung surfactant and can destabilize the alveoli, allowing them to collapse and thus not be available for breathing.

The microbes causing sepsis leading to ARDS vary widely in type and geographic distribution. In developed countries, bacterial infections are the most common, often with organisms partially or highly resistant to antibiotics that are common in hospital environments. Viruses that cause pneumonias can cause ARDS. In fact, most of the deaths in the severe acute respiratory syndrome (SARS) and H1N1 influenza epidemics were due to ARDS.

How is it prevented, treated, and managed?

Prevention, treatment, staying healthy, prognosis

Prevention of ARDS can be accomplished by preventing the infections and injuries that cause it. Even if trauma or infection cannot be prevented, early aggressive treatment may avert ARDS. Promptly hydrating persons in shock or administering antibiotics to persons with pneumonia may correct the underlying process enough to prevent ARDS from developing.

Once ARDS develops, the management of these patients consists of appropriate treatment of the underlying or causative illness, excellent supportive care, and prevention of complications. Appropriate treatment of an underlying infection is particularly important and consists of identifying the causative organism as best as possible and draining any abscesses, as well as giving antibiotics.

The care of the critically ill patient is highly complex because of the severity of the patient's illness, the combination of diseases and organ failures and their interactions, and the rapidity of changes in the patient's condition.

Mechanical ventilation is a key component of good supportive care. The ventilator must be set to deliver enough air to make sure the patient's oxygen level is adequate. Positive end-expiratory pressure (PEEP) is applied to each breath to keep alveoli open, and a host of other adjustments are made to keep

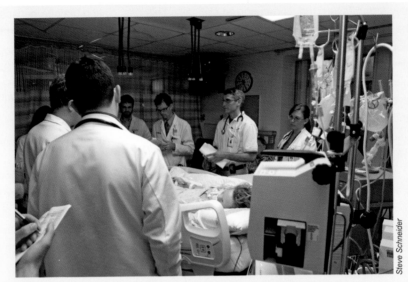

An intensive care unit is a busy and complicated place, where patients are comprehensively monitored, and interventions take place quickly. Improvements in how patients are cared for in these units are quite likely to be responsible for the better outcomes in acute respiratory distress syndrome

the patient alive without causing harm to the lungs or the rest of the body. The use of small breaths from the ventilator avoids further injury and is particularly important.

Fluid management is complex in ARDS because the lungs are flooding while the patient often does not have enough blood volume to maintain an adequate blood pressure. Although sedative and pain relief medications are essential, too much sedation can keep the patient on the ventilator longer than necessary and cause delirium and lack of cooperation. Medicines that are eliminated by the liver or kidney may accumulate and interact if these organs are dysfunctional. Other treatments may also cause harm. The mere presence of a tube in the trachea to deliver the ventilation is associated with increased risk of pneumonia. One of the goals is also to reduce patient discomfort related to the tubes, blood drawing, alarms, and frequent nursing checks.

A critical decision for an improving patient is when to remove the mechanical ventilation. The longer a patient remains on the ventilator, the greater the chance of complications, including airway injury from the tube and pneumonia. Once the patient's ventilation requirements have decreased to a predetermined level, the patient is given a daily trial of breathing on his or her own (spontaneous breathing trial) to see if breathing can comfortably continue and adequate oxygenation can be maintained.

The death rate associated with ARDS is high, with overall mortality between 30 and 40 percent. Once a patient survives the acute episode of ARDS, his or her lung function gradually improves over the next six months to a year, with eventual return to normal or near-normal lung function in nearly all cases. An occasional patient is left with significant scarring and lower than normal lung volumes.

Despite normal lung function in nearly all survivors, in self-assessments, these patients frequently rate their quality of life as impaired. Recent studies of ARDS survivors have found psychological problems, including higher than expected rates of depression and post-traumatic stress disorder, neurocognitive problems that are usually relatively mild in degree and improve over years, and neuromuscular weakness. The causes of these problems and how best to prevent and treat them are subjects of intense research interest.

Are we making a difference?

Research past, present, and future

Although the mortality related to ARDS is high, it has substantially improved in recent years. This decline in the death rate started before any specific treatment had been shown to be beneficial for ARDS and was likely related to improvements in critical care medicine and management of these patients.

A great deal has been learned about the inflammatory process and how fluids are handled in the lung, but inflammation is a highly complex process, with new molecules and pathways—and their cellular interactions—being discovered regularly. Several trials have tested intervention in the inflammatory process, but none have shown substantial benefit.

Considerable interest exists in whether genetic makeup affects the development of ARDS, but the research in this area is in its early stages. Some gene mutations have been shown to be associated with an increased risk of ARDS development, but for the overwhelming majority of cases of ARDS, no specific genetic profile has been identified. Interest remains high because of the clinical observation that while two patients may share similar characteristics and have the same disease, one may develop ARDS and the other may not.

Life-saving mechanical ventilation can itself result in further injury to the already-injured lungs of patients with ARDS. At times this ventilator-induced lung injury can result in worse and more permanent damage than that produced by ARDS itself. The National Institutes of Health sponsored the ARDS Clinical Network (commonly called *ARDSnet*) to carry out studies on patients with ARDS in the intensive care unit (ICU). One study published in 2000 showed that patients given smaller ventilator breaths had significantly higher survival than patients with conventional treatment (3). It also showed that the use of large breaths resulted in ongoing inflammation that traveled beyond the lungs. New modes of "lung protective ventilation" have been developed. The value of PEEP has been established in several studies, although determining the best level of PEEP for an individual patient remains an elusive goal.

Studies have shown that daily spontaneous breathing trials (without the ventilator's help) resulted in fewer days on the ventilator. To do the trials, it was necessary to stop sedation, which has also been shown to be beneficial. A simple method to help minimize aspiration and reduce the risk of developing pneumonia is to raise the head of the bed to between 30 and 45 degrees.

An ARDSnet study of ICU patients showed that a more conservative fluid administration strategy—initiated after adequate fluid intake was ensured—resulted in less time on mechanical ventilation and less time in the ICU. Other advances are being made and are tied closely to the management of patients in the intensive care unit.

What we need to cure or eliminate ARDS

Although it is not realistic to speak of cure when considering a form of injury, the two factors most likely to reduce the burden of ARDS are continued improvement in the care of patients in the ICU and breakthroughs in the understanding of the inflammatory process that result in new therapies. Technologies to better monitor and treat ARDS patients and evaluation of current procedures have resulted in past gains and are likely to continue to steadily increase patient care outcome. Gains from understanding the inflammatory process are long-term goals that are likely to help treat patients with ARDS and with many other diseases in which inflammation plays a part.

References

1. Bernard GR, Artigas A, Brigham KL, Carlet J, Falke K, Hudson L, Lamy M, Legall JR, Morris A, Spragg R. The American-European Consensus Conference on ARDS. Definitions, mechanisms, relevant outcomes, and clinical trial coordination. *Am J Respir Crit Care Med* 1994;149:818–824.
2. Rubenfeld GD, Caldwell E, Peabody E, Weaver J, Martin DP, Neff M, Stern EJ, Hudson LD. Incidence and outcomes of acute lung injury. *N Engl J Med* 2005;353:1685–1693.
3. The Acute Respiratory Distress Syndrome Network. Ventilation with lower tidal volumes as compared with traditional tidal volumes for acute lung injury and the acute respiratory distress syndrome. *N Engl J Med* 2000;342:1301–1308.

Web sites of interest

National Heart, Lung, and Blood Institute
www.nhlbi.nih.gov/health/dci/Diseases/Ards/Ards_WhatIs.html

ARDS Foundation
www.ardsil.com

ARDS Support Center
www.ards.org

National Heart, Lung, and Blood Institute ARDS Network (ARDSNet)
www.ardsnet.org

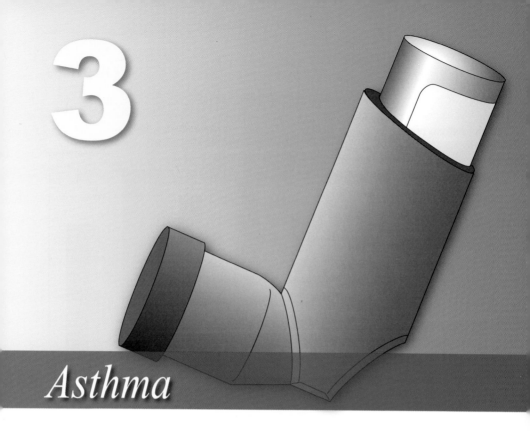

3

Asthma

Asthma is a common but complex disease of the pulmonary airways (trachea, bronchi, and bronchioles) that is characterized by difficulties getting air in and out of the lungs (variable airflow obstruction), environmental triggers causing breathlessness (airway hyperresponsiveness), and cellular inflammation.

Whom does it affect?

Epidemiology, prevalence, economic burden, vulnerable populations

Epidemiological studies have established features of asthma and provided insight into many of its characteristics, including the age of onset, sex distribution, risk factors, and long-term consequences. The International Study of Asthma and Allergies in Childhood (ISAAC) surveyed nearly 200,000 children six to seven years old and over 300,000 children 13 to 14 years old in more than 50 countries (1). The results from this survey found the prevalence of asthma to be over 10 percent in some countries, including the United Kingdom, New Zealand, Australia, Costa Rica, the United States, and Brazil. In contrast, in other countries, like China, the prevalence of asthma is slightly over 5 percent. In recent years, some countries and locales have demonstrated a near doubling in the prevalence of asthma.

Asthma prevalence by age, gender, and race in the United States, 2006

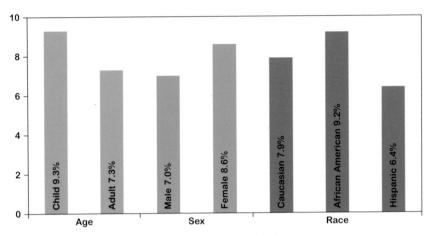

Asthma poses a greater risk for children, women, and African Americans.
National Health Interview Survey, National Center for Health Statistics, Centers for Disease Control and Prevention.

From these and other surveys, it is apparent that asthma prevalence is influenced by a variety of factors (2,3). First, the presence of asthma is greatest in the more "westernized" areas of the world—the Americas, Europe, and Australia. Second, as more countries shift their lifestyle to a more western pattern of living (which includes fewer severe infections early in life, greater use of antibiotics, more processed foods, and a shift from rural to urban living) the prevalence of asthma increases. Finally, in countries with a less western lifestyle, the prevalence of asthma is low and remains at this level until such societal changes occur. These data suggest that factors associated with a western lifestyle are associated with a greater risk or frequency of asthma (2). These epidemiological changes led to the development of the "hygiene hypothesis," which proposes that a "cleaner" environment shifts the immune response toward the development of allergies and asthma (4).

In the United States, the prevalence of asthma has followed the increase seen worldwide over the past two decades (5). From 1980 to the late 1990s, the prevalence of asthma doubled, with rates of 6 percent in children and more than 4 percent in adults. Prevalence assessments are dependent on how the asthma is identified. For example, when asthma is characterized as an "attack," the prevalence is less than 4 percent. If the question asked is, "Have you had asthma in your lifetime?" over 10 percent of respondents will answer yes, which more accurately reflects the at-risk population. By any measure, asthma is the most common pulmonary disease in children.

Individual risk factors for asthma include a family history of asthma or allergies, a mother who smokes, being raised in an urban environment, early development of eczema (atopic dermatitis), and the appearance of environmental allergies (6). For the at-risk child, certain environmental allergens—house dust mites, cockroaches, and molds such as *Alternaria*—are most likely to be important to the development of asthma. The contribution of animal dander from dogs and cats is undergoing re-evaluation, with some evidence saying that, depending on the age of exposure, the presence of dogs, more so than cats, protects against the development of asthma.

These epidemiological observations have also indicated that two components are necessary for asthma to develop: genetic and environmental factors. Both risks are needed: the right genes and the right environment. One without the other is not sufficient to lead to the expression of asthma.

In adolescence, a number of changes may occur in patients with asthma. First, some previously symptomatic patients will have a remission of their disease; whether it is "permanent" is not clear, nor is it known which patients are likely to experience this loss of symptoms. Second, some patients develop asthma at this time of their life; the factors associated with later onset are not clear. Third, there is a shift in the sex prevalence in the teen years, with adolescent girls or women more likely to have asthma than their male counterparts (7).

The burden of asthma is also significant and felt at many levels—personal, family, and societal. The costs of medications alone for this common and chronic disease can be $3,000 to $4,000 per patient annually. Asthma remains the number one cause of admission to the hospital for children, which has significant costs (8,9). Severe episodes of asthma that lead to hospitalization occur seasonally, with September and October the most common months, probably owing to cold viruses entering the community when children return to school. Asthma has other costs, including missed time from school of approximately 12.8 million days per year in the United States (10). Costs associated with asthma also arise in indirect ways, such as family members who need to miss work to obtain treatment for asthma, especially for children. In the United States, the annual cost of asthma exceeds $19 billion per year.

CASE STUDY

A 25-year-old woman had lifelong asthma. Coughing and wheezing began with a cold when she was two years old. She was initially diagnosed with bronchitis, but antibiotics were not effective. By age five, she had environmental allergies, including reactions to house dust mites and cats. She missed about two weeks of school per year, usually following a cold that led to an asthma episode. Systemic corticosteroids (prednisone) were required three or four times per year, along with the use of daily inhaled corticosteroids.

As a teenager, her symptoms remitted. Her need for medications lessened, prednisone bursts were less than one per year, and her ability to participate in physical activity was normal. However, at age 21, she developed a severe upper respiratory infection, which led to sinusitis and reoccurrence of her asthma. Her symptoms intensified; an emergency room visit was needed for an acute episode of breathlessness and wheezing. Eventually, a prolonged course of prednisone was required to achieve control of her asthma. She was able to stop prednisone and use only inhaled corticosteroids and a long-acting beta-agonist, but she continued to experience chest tightness, awoke at night about once per week, and had limitation to exercise. If she forgot to take her medications, asthma symptoms reappeared, which provided daily reminders of her disease.

Comment

The patient described in this case illustrates the natural history of asthma, which has provided essential clues to the mechanisms of the disease, enhanced diagnostic approaches, and led to improved and more specific treatments. For example, in most patients, asthma begins in the first six years of life. Early episodes of wheezing are frequently in association with viral respiratory infections, the most predominant of which are common cold viruses (rhinoviruses). For many children, these wheezing episodes become fewer and fewer as they grow older. However, many patients have progression of their symptoms, in terms of severity and persistence, with the development of respiratory allergies or infections.

What are we learning about asthma?

Pathophysiology, causes: genetic, environment, microbes

The past 15 to 20 years have seen progress in understanding the basic mechanisms of asthma, earlier recognition and treatment, and more effective and safe medications for asthma, with important new discoveries made on a yearly basis.

In addition to the appreciation of environmental and genetic factors involved in the expression of asthma, our understanding of the processes in the lung that lead to asthma and of the clinical manifestations has increased dramatically. Three decades

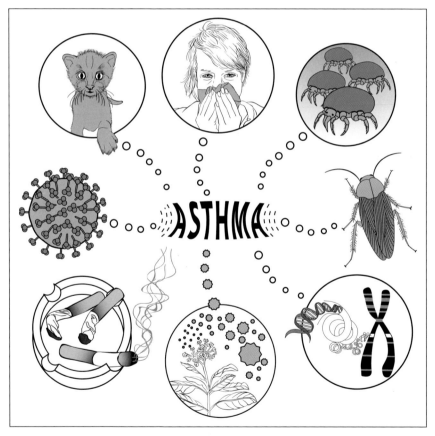

Among the best-know instigators and triggers of asthma are (starting at the bottom and going clockwise) pollens, cigarette smoke, respiratory viruses, pet dander, colds and allergies, house dust mites, cockroaches, and a genetic predisposition.

ago, asthma was considered a "bronchospastic" disease of airways. That is, it was thought that asthma consisted of the airway smooth muscles contracting too easily and too frequently. At that time, the primary treatment was bronchodilators, which were designed to relax the contracted airway muscle in order to reduce the bronchospasm and wheezing. Bronchodilators are still needed to treat asthma and are effective, but they address only one component of the disease.

Although asthma has been known to be a chronic disease, the driving elements of its persistence have been unclear. It is now well recognized that airway inflammation is an essential feature of asthma and is present on a chronic basis, but it will "wax and wane" to make asthma improve or worsen. Airway inflammation is also a key target to successful treatment of asthma.

It is also now appreciated that inflammation in asthma is complex and involves many different cells and mediators (11). For example, white blood cells, mast cells, airway lining cells (epithelium), smooth muscle, mucous glands, and nerves are involved. Each of these cells produces many chemical mediators that interact to promote and induce the inflammatory response. The overall consequence of inflammation is multi-factorial, with narrowing of the airways, increased likelihood of bronchospasm (hyperresponsiveness), and persistence of asthma.

Airway inflammation can be provoked by allergic reactions, viral respiratory infections, environmental material, and occupational exposures. The most effective remedy is avoidance, where and when possible. However, this approach is not always possible because of the ubiquitous nature of many environmental exposures.

How is it prevented, treated, and managed?

Prevention, treatment, staying healthy, prognosis

Asthma can begin at any age in life, but most commonly, onset occurs in children younger than six years of age. For these patients, asthma is often associated with hay fever (allergic rhinitis) and eczema (atopic dermatitis). For these patients, environment allergens play a large and significant role in the onset of disease and persistence of symptoms. Asthma can also begin in adulthood. In this setting, allergic diseases are usually not a major factor, but the disease is more severe, with co-existing sinusitis a frequent finding (7,11).

The diagnosis of asthma, particularly in children, is primarily based upon symptoms of cough, wheeze, and shortness of breath in the presence of other

Web sites of interest

National Heart, Lung, and Blood Institute
Guidelines for the Diagnosis and Management of Asthma
www.nhlbi.nih.gov/guidelines/asthma/asthgdln.htm

Medline Plus links to many resources
www.nlm.nih.gov/medlineplus/asthma.html

Asthma and Allergy Foundation of America
www.aafa.org/

The Environment Protection Agency's Asthma Program
www.epa.gov/asthma

Centers for Disease Control and Prevention Asthma Information
www.cdc.gov/ASTHMA

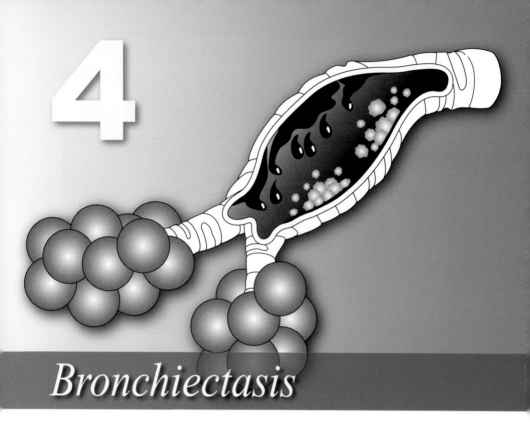

Bronchiectasis

Bronchiectasis is an abnormal, chronic enlargement of the bronchi, the passageways from the trachea to the alveoli that are the air-exchanging parts of the lungs. Bronchiectasis generally occurs as a result of infection, although non-infectious factors may contribute to the development of this condition. Accompanying the enlargement of the bronchi is their decreased ability to clear secretions. Failure to clear secretions allows microbes and particles to collect in them, which leads to more secretions and inflammation that further damage the airways, causing more dilation in a vicious cycle.

Bronchiectasis may occur in a single portion of the lung (localized) or throughout the lungs (diffuse) and is the major lung abnormality of cystic fibrosis. It may have several different contributing factors, such as abnormal cilia, and its course may vary greatly from causing no symptoms to causing death.

Whom does it affect?

Epidemiology, prevalence, economic burden, vulnerable populations

The prevalence of bronchiectasis is unknown largely because the symptoms are variable and the diagnosis is often not made. In the pre-antibiotic era, it was estimated to be as common as or more common than tuberculosis and to be

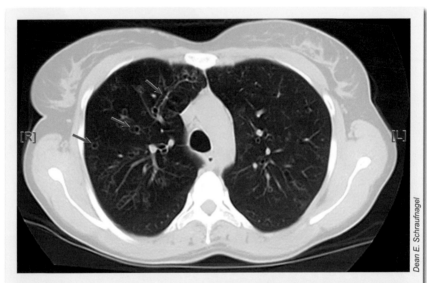

This computed tomographic (CT) image of the lungs shows dilation of the bronchi characteristic of bronchiectasis (arrows). The large white structure in the center is the aorta and the darker areas are normal lung.

Dean E. Schraufnagel

present in 92 percent of cases of chronic bronchitis (1). It occurs in every age group and, in the pre-antibiotic era, it most often began in childhood (1). Among all ages, it has been estimated that about 25 people per 100,000 have bronchiectasis, but this number increases to 272 per 100,000 for those over 74 years old (2). However, these statistics were derived from insurance data, which is likely to grossly underestimate its true occurrence. Cases of bronchiectasis are more common in women than men, especially when it is of unknown cause.

A wide range of causes of bronchiectasis has been reported in adults, but for more than half of the cases, there is no known cause or association. It is estimated that between 30 and 35 percent of cases follow a lung infection that damages the bronchi for the first time (3). In addition to bacterial pneumonia, other infections, such as whooping cough (pertussis) or tuberculosis, may cause the bronchial damage. Although the inciting infections are usually severe, bronchiectasis can also occur with minimal or silent infections. This is often the case when the inciting infection is caused by nontuberculous mycobacteria (see Chapter 12).

Individuals with an inadequate immune system are at increased risk for chronic bronchial infections, which can damage airways and set up conditions

Bronchiectasis

Prevalence of Bronchiectasis

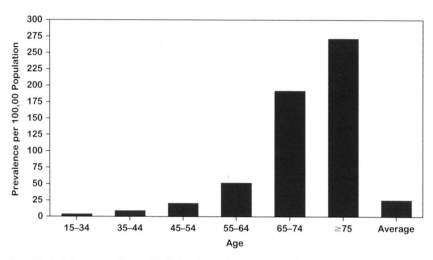

Bronchiectasis increases with age. It is likely to be much more common than reported here because it is not usually detected, reported, or treated (2).

for bronchiectasis. Persons who fail to produce antibodies, a condition that can be congenital or acquired, commonly develop bronchiectasis. Other immune deficiency states are also associated with bronchiectasis.

The economic burden attributed to bronchiectasis is great, in part, because it is a chronic disease that may require frequent medical visits, antibiotics, hospitalizations, and chest physiotherapy in order to minimize the risk of recurrent infections and progressive disease. In 2001, it was estimated that the annual medical cost of care for persons in the United States with bronchiectasis was $13,244, which is greater than the annual cost for many other chronic diseases, such as heart disease ($12,000) and COPD ($11,000 to $13,000) (2). If there are over 110,000 persons in the United States with bronchiectasis, expenditures for medical care are estimated to be greater than $1.4 billion annually.

For patients who have airway infections resistant to oral antibiotics, the burden is much greater. Intravenous antibiotics complicate care greatly because hospitalization or home monitoring is required. Treatment for these patients includes placement of a central venous catheter, coordination of the doses of drugs that often must be given multiple times per day, regular blood tests to monitor for side effects, and measurement of blood levels of the antibiotic for many days, steps that become expensive and disrupt patients' lives.

CASE STUDY

A 57-year-old woman was referred to a pulmonologist for worsening cough and sputum production over nearly two years. A nonsmoker, she appeared thin but not in distress and had no other significant medical problems. Additional symptoms included shortness of breath and fatigue. Her primary care physician had treated her with antibiotics for bronchitis six times over the previous 18 months. She had no heartburn, acid reflux, choking, or sinus symptoms. There was no systemic inflammatory disease, history of tuberculosis, or other chest infections, such as whooping cough. She had no family history of lung disease. A chest radiograph showed dilated airways in several areas that were confirmed by a chest computed tomography (CT) scan. Blood tests, including antibody (immunoglobulin) levels, were normal. Pulmonary function testing demonstrated a decrease in lung capacity with mild airflow obstruction that significantly improved with an inhaled bronchodilator. Sputum collected for bacterial culture grew the bacteria Pseudomonas aeruginosa. *Bronchiectasis was diagnosed, and the patient began a treatment program that included a bronchodilator, a mucus-clearance device, chest physiotherapy, antibiotics, and a regular exercise program. Over the next 12 months, her symptoms improved dramatically, although they did not resolve completely. She regained her energy and was able to resume her normal lifestyle that included recreational activities, such as golfing, while continuing with her pulmonary treatment program.*

Comment

This case study represents several common features of bronchiectasis. The diagnosis of bronchiectasis is frequently delayed for months or years, often with symptoms misdiagnosed as bronchitis, asthma, or recurrent pneumonia. Symptoms are often downplayed by both the patient and physician. Once diagnosed, bronchiectasis requires a health maintenance program with intermittent treatment of airway infections. This program is usually tailored to the patient's symptoms and can range from occasional follow-up to frequent hospitalizations for intensive treatment. Chest radiographs or CT scans allow visualization of the dilated bronchi and can also diagnose pneumonia, which is a recognized complication. Pulmonary function tests demonstrate impairment of lung function when present.

Bronchiectasis

What are we learning about the disease?

Pathophysiology, causes: genetic, environment, microbes

The respiratory tract is lined with cells that contain cilia, hair-like structures that stick into the mucous layer that lines the airways and beat to propel the mucus out of the lungs. Mucus traps bacteria and particles, and mucociliary clearance is an important defense mechanism for the bronchial tubes. It is not surprising that a variety of problems of cilia are associated with bronchiectasis. Ciliated cells also line the inner surface of the nose and sinuses, which are part of the respiratory tract. Ciliary disorders usually, therefore, also are associated with sinus infections. Sinus disease is common in bronchiectasis even when a ciliary defect is not known.

Almost any cause of significant bronchial injury can lead to bronchiectasis. Several auto-immune diseases, such as rheumatoid arthritis or Sjögren's syndrome, can cause bronchiectasis. Aspiration of oral contents can be particularly damaging. Gastroesophageal reflux disease (GERD) with gastric aspiration may contribute as well. Even obstruction of the airway by an inhaled peanut or other

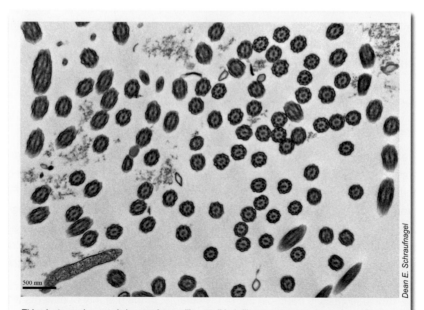

This electron microscopic image shows cilia, small hair-like structures on the surface of cells in the airways. Ciliary defects are associated with bronchiectasis. Cilia move mucus out of the lung. About 200 cilia are present on the surface of each cell, and more than 250 genes are responsible for their proper functioning.

Dean E. Schraufnagel

foreign body can set up conditions for bronchiectasis by blocking drainage of normal mucus. Other impairments in the bronchial structure or mucociliary clearance can also cause it. For example, thick mucus can be retained in bronchi in patients with asthma. If the mucus becomes infected by a common fungus, *Aspergillus*, an intense inflammation can ensue. The inflammation can damage the airway and result in bronchiectasis.

In addition to cystic fibrosis, inherited conditions like immotile ciliary syndrome and alpha-1 antitrypsin deficiency may lead to bronchiectasis. A rare condition called *Ehlers-Danlos syndrome* causes lax supporting tissue in and around the airway that, under certain circumstances, can be associated with bronchiectasis. Bronchiectasis can also occur in a variety of rare genetic defects of the immune system.

Infection by environmental nontuberculous mycobacteria (see Chapter 12) is also being recognized and treated, with significant improvement in patients' quality of life. These ubiquitous bacteria are in the same family as *Mycobacterium tuberculosis* but are not contagious. They have a propensity to live in the secretions of patients with bronchiectasis. Most mycobacterial infections can be treated, but they require many months or even years of medication. Certain bacteria such as *Pseudomonas* and other drug-resistant organisms may be difficult to treat and require inhaled or intravenous antibiotics.

How is it prevented, treated, and managed?

Prevention, treatment, staying healthy, prognosis

Prevention of bronchiectasis is difficult because the risk for developing it is generally not known before the diagnosis. However, if a cause is known and can be corrected, that becomes the highest priority in managing bronchiectasis. For example, correcting a lack of antibodies (agammaglobulinemia) or removing a bronchial obstruction may "cure" the bronchiectasis. If other causative or aggravating conditions are present, they should be treated. For example, aspiration should be prevented, and infectious and other associated inflammatory disorders generally should be treated.

Bronchiectasis is treatable but rarely curable. In the majority of patients with bronchiectasis, there are strategies for preventing or slowing its progression. The two most important elements of these strategies are clearance of airway secretions and prompt treatment of lung infections. Retained secretions in the airway make a favorable environment for bacteria to flourish, resulting in the cycle of infection, airway inflammation, airway injury with further enlargement, and more retained secretions. Untreated, this cycle of infection, inflammation, and injury often results in progressive symptoms and loss of lung function. In one study, poor prognosis was correlated with decreased activity and quality of life, chronic *Pseudomonas aeruginosa* infection, and poor pulmonary function tests (4).

General self-care techniques are an important part of bronchiectasis treatment. These techniques include such infection prevention methods as proper hand washing, covering the mouth when coughing, and appropriate vaccinations. Regular aerobic activity, a balanced diet, and avoidance of all tobacco products are also important.

As bronchiectasis advances, symptoms are more frequent and severe, and eradication of the infection and secretions becomes more difficult. The goal of therapy remains to minimize symptoms, prevent loss of lung function, and preserve quality of life.

Keeping airways clear of secretions helps break the infection, inflammation, and injury cycle and is a key for successful management of patients with bronchiectasis. For those patients that do not produce sputum ("dry bronchiectasis"), little is needed to do to keep airways clear. In these patients, chronic infection is uncommon.

Most patients with bronchiectasis produce from a teaspoon to over a cup of sputum per day. Techniques for clearing retained secretions vary greatly. In some instances, regular exercise is sufficient to mobilize and clear them. Chest percussion with or without postural drainage is often first tried to raise sputum. Several medical devices are marketed for this purpose. These may be simple handheld instruments that vibrate air in the airway or more complicated chest-wall vibrating devices. The vibration may "shake loose" thick mucus, but not all techniques work for every patient, and a trial-and-error approach is usually required to find the most effective regimen for a specific patient. Lack of hydration may thicken sputum, so drinking plenty of fluids is generally recommended.

Airway inflammation with asthmatic-like reactions is often present in bronchiectatic airways and most often should be treated with asthma medications, such as inhaled bronchodilators or inhaled corticosteroids. Bronchodilators relax airway muscles and may enhance mucous clearance. Inhaled corticosteroids reduce inflammation and may be beneficial in select patients. Nebulized concentrated salt solution (hypertonic saline) affords enhanced secretion clearance in cystic fibrosis patients, but its benefit to other patients with bronchiectasis remains unproven.

Finally, a small subgroup of patients with localized bronchiectasis may benefit from surgical resection of the affected area of the lung. This procedure is most often done if the lung segment is a site of substantial bleeding, bronchial obstruction, or recurrent infection.

Are we making a difference?

Research past, present, and future

Since the first description of bronchiectasis by René Laënnec in the early 1800s, knowledge has been gained about the natural history, the characteristics of different bacteria, and the structure and physiology of the cells of the airways. Antibiotics have transformed bronchiectasis from a common sequela of pneumonia to an uncommon condition. They have also greatly improved the quality of life of these patients.

The discovery of the gene that causes cystic fibrosis in 1989 allowed more detailed knowledge of the biology of the cells of the airway, the transport of water and salts into the mucus, and the character of the sputum, although treatments for cystic fibrosis do not necessarily translate into the care of patients with bronchiectasis without cystic fibrosis.

Bronchiectasis is associated with cellular and molecular defects and adverse events that result in airway injury, mucus stagnation, and infection. Research has advanced the knowledge of each of these areas. More is being learned about who gets bronchiectasis. The complexity of ciliated cells and other bronchial lining cells is being recognized.

The slimy material that collects at the bottom of standing water is called a biofilm. Biofilms are usually made up of a community of many different bacteria; some bacteria produce the slimy material and other bacteria use it for their advantage. In humans, dental plaque is an example of a biofilm. Biofilms also occur in the airways of patients with bronchiectasis. If one species of bacteria produces a substance that inactivates an antibiotic, all the other organisms in the biofilm benefit.

Biofilm material forms a submicroscopic netlike mesh that may prevent the body's immune cells from engulfing and destroying the bacteria. The bacteria of the biofilm communicate to inform each other about the concentration of bacteria. The communications may signal the bacteria to grow if conditions are favorable, or to reduce activity if conditions are not. A change in activity of the bacteria could irritate the bronchial lining cells and set off an episode of cough, sputum, and breathlessness.

As more is being learned about biofilms, new agents are being developed that can block the inter-bacterial communication. Although antibiotics and secretion clearance have led to stabilization of bronchiectasis in most patients, better antibiotics are being developed to allow oral medications and nebulized solutions to replace intravenous medicines to treat exacerbations of bronchiectasis.

A national non-cystic fibrosis bronchiectasis registry has been established to better define the patients and the infections they get. This registry has been modeled after the one for cystic fibrosis patients that was established many years ago. Genetic studies, which would investigate predisposing factors, should open new doors to study the cells and molecules that fail to protect against bronchiectasis as well as to alert persons who might be at increased risk for the disease.

What we need to cure and eliminate bronchiectasis

Bronchiectasis is almost certainly less frequent and severe today than it was in the preantibiotic era. Treatment of pneumonia with antibiotics has reduced cases of bronchiectasis, a common sequelia. Development of antibiotics that are easier to deliver and more effective should further reduce its burden. The next steps toward eliminating bronchiectasis require better understanding of the basic mechanisms of the disease, the organisms involved, biofilms, and how the lung damage is perpetuated. Research on nontuberculous mycobacteria, their relation to the mucus layer, and susceptibility to new antibiotics will likely help control this group of pathogens. Clinical trials need to be done to determine when, which, and how long antibiotics should be given. Lastly, awareness leading to more prompt diagnosis and treatment of both bronchiectasis and its underlying conditions is essential to reduce and control this disease.

References

1. Scarlett EP. Bronchiectasis (A review). *Can Med Assoc J* 1946; 54:275–283.
2. O'Donnell AE. Bronchiectasis. *Chest* 2008;134:815–823
3. Weycker D, Edelsberg J, Oster G, Tino G. Prevalence and economic burden of bronchiectasis. *Clin Pulm Med* 2005;12:205–209.
4. Loebinger MR, Wells AU, Hansell DM, Chinyanganya N, Devaraj A, Meister M, Wilson R. Mortality in bronchiectasis: a long-term study assessing the factors influencing survival. *Eur Respir J* 2009; 34:843–849.

Web sites of interest

Bronchiectasis Research Registry
www.cscc.unc.edu/bron

National Heart, Lung, and Blood Institute
Diseases and Conditions Index
www.nhlbi.nih.gov/health/dci/index.html

Nontuberculous Mycobacteria Info & Research, Inc.
http://ntminfo.org

Cystic Fibrosis Foundation
www.cff.org

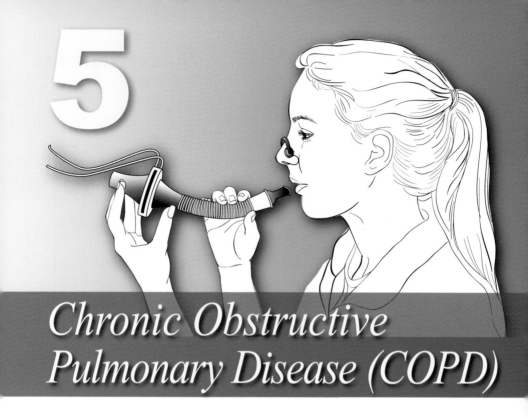

Chronic Obstructive Pulmonary Disease (COPD)

Chronic obstructive pulmonary disease (COPD) is an umbrella term for conditions, including chronic bronchitis and emphysema, that impede the flow of air in the bronchi and trachea. COPD is the fourth-leading cause of death in the United States and is a major cause of sickness. It is currently the fifth-leading cause of death worldwide, but the World Health Organization projects it will become the third-leading cause by 2030 (1). COPD is both preventable and treatable.

International organizations have more specifically defined COPD as "a disease state characterized by airflow limitation that is not fully reversible. The airflow limitation is usually both progressive and associated with an abnormal inflammatory response of the lungs to noxious particles or gases."

Whom does it affect?

Definition, epidemiology, prevalence, economic burden, and vulnerable populations

Chronic obstructive pulmonary disease is diagnosed using a medical device called a spirometer, which measures air volume and flow, the main components of common clinical breathing tests (pulmonary function tests). The measurement

Rate of COPD deaths by state, per 100,000 population

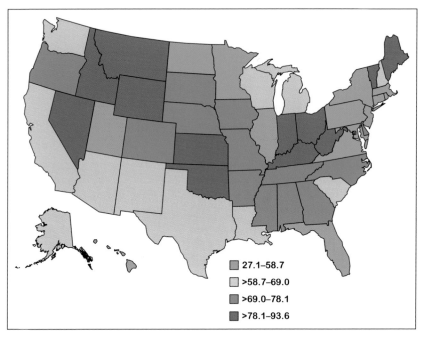

27.1–58.7
>58.7–69.0
>69.0–78.1
>78.1–93.6

Deaths from COPD vary by state, which may reflect differences in smoking, diagnosis, or treatment.
Centers for Disease Control and Prevention. *National Vital Statistics System.* Atlanta: 2005.

of the forced expired volume of air in one second (FEV_1) as a percentage of the total amount of air that can be forcefully exhaled (forced vital capacity or FVC) is the main functional way of defining COPD. An FEV_1/FVC ratio less than 0.70 after a patient is given a bronchodilator usually indicates that he or she has COPD. A progressive disease, COPD is widely recognized as having four stages of severity. At its most severe stage, the FEV_1 is less than 30 percent of normal (2).

COPD is a common chronic disease. Most estimates of COPD put its prevalence in the adult population in the 5 to 10 percent range, although these estimates vary by the specific criteria used. The Third National Health and Nutrition Examination Survey (NHANES III) data—the most recent U.S. survey that included spirometry—showed a prevalence of COPD in adults of 6.8 percent (1). Over 50 percent of people with evidence of COPD, though, have never been

Estimated number of men and women hospitalized for COPD

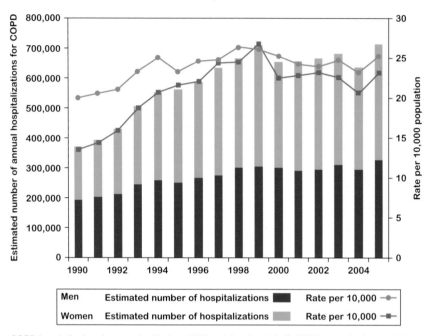

COPD hospitalizations increased until about 2000 and then leveled off. COPD rates shadow smoking rates with a delay of several years. DeFrances CJ, Hall MJ, for the Division of Health Care Statistics. 2005 National Hospital Discharge Survey. Hyattsville, MD: 2007.

diagnosed with disease. This proportion is even higher among people with mild disease, which is most amenable to intervention (3).

COPD is responsible for about 700,000 hospitalizations annually in the United States. In recent years, the hospitalization rate among women has increased and is now similar to the rate among men. In 2005, more than 126,000 adults in the United States died from COPD (4). Age-adjusted mortality rates varied dramatically by state, from a low of 27.1 per 100,000 in Hawaii to a high of 93.6 per 100,000 in Oklahoma.

COPD has an enormous financial burden, with estimated direct medical costs in 1993 of $14.7 billion. The estimated indirect cost related to morbidity (loss of work time and productivity) and premature mortality is an additional $9.2 billion, for a total of $23.9 billion annually. By 2002, this cost was estimated at $32.1 billion annually (1).

CASE STUDY

A 52-year-old woman sought medical attention for increasing shortness of breath on exertion for over two years. She used to walk 9 holes of golf with her women's group every Wednesday, but over the last year she has had to use a golf cart. She has attributed this change to getting old. She was told three years earlier that she had "a touch of asthma" and was given an inhaler to use when she was symptomatic. In the last six months, she had three trips to the emergency department for "acute bronchitis." She had smoked for about 15 years, but stopped 20 years ago. Spirometry showed an FEV_1 of 62 percent of that predicted and an FEV_1/FVC of 0.58.

Comment

This case highlights several typical features of COPD. First, it is becoming increasingly common among women, and women are more likely to be misdiagnosed (5). Second, people with COPD are told they have asthma or another respiratory disease. Third, the symptoms can occur long after a person has stopped smoking, and, in some cases, in the absence of a smoking history altogether. People often attribute their breathing problems to other causes, and they may feel that once they have stopped smoking they will no longer suffer its consequences.

What we are learning about the disease

Pathophysiology, causes: genetic, environment, microbes

COPD comprises a collection of different processes, including chronic or recurrent bronchitis, emphysema, and airway responsiveness that contribute to the disease. The most important risk factor for COPD in the United States is cigarette smoking. Other factors, including occupational or environmental exposures to dusts, gases, vapors, biomass smoke, malnutrition, early life infections, recurrent respiratory infections, genetic predisposition, increased airways responsiveness, and asthma may be important in many individuals (3).

Chronic or recurrent bronchitis is a major component of COPD. It consists of bouts of increased cough and sputum production that can occur frequently. The attacks may be related to an acute bacterial or viral infection or a chronic

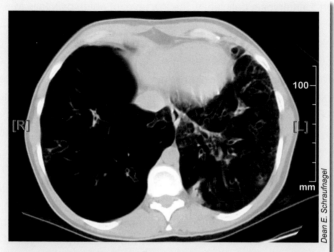

This computed tomography (CT) scan shows emphysema on the right (R), where most of the lung tissue is replaced by large spaces of air. The left side (L) has bronchitis and bronchiectasis—dilated bronchi with thickened walls. This image would be characteristic of alpha-1 antitrypsin deficiency, although this patient did not have it.

process that has permanently damaged the airways, known as bronchiectasis. While most people have had an episode of bronchitis at some point in their life, recurrent episodes (typically two to three per year) are frequently observed in COPD.

Emphysema, another component of COPD, entails the destruction of alveoli (air sacs) in the lungs, impairing their ability to bring oxygen into the body and eliminate carbon dioxide.

The best known genetic risk factor for COPD is alpha-1 antitrypsin deficiency. Alpha-1 antitrypsin is a special protein that protects the lungs from enzymes known as proteases. The body's white blood cells seek out and destroy bacteria and viruses trying to invade the lungs. They kill the microbes by releasing enzymes and other toxic products that, in addition to killing the organisms, can damage the lungs. Alpha-1 antitrypsin quickly inactivates the enzymes produced by these white cells, protecting the lung from damage. In individuals with alpha-1 antitrypsin deficiency, the low level of antitrypsin fails to protect the lungs from enzymatic tissue damage. This is a major cause of COPD in patients with alpha-1 antitrypsin deficiency. There are approximately 100,000 people in the United States who are deficient in alpha-1 antitrypsin because of a genetic defect. These patients can develop lung disease even in the absence of cigarette smoking, although smoking increases their chances of developing it.

COPD is also increasingly associated with other diseases, such as pneumonia, hypertension, heart failure, forms of heart disease, lung vascular disease, cancer, osteoporosis, and depression.

Although the role of environmental factors like cigarette smoke in the causation of COPD is well established, the mechanisms linking the exposure to the disease at the cellular level are still poorly understood. For instance, it is known that a characteristic form of inflammation involving a type of white blood cell (neutrophilic leukocytes) is associated with the structural changes of the lung that are found in chronic bronchitis and emphysema. However, the critical biological pathways remain elusive. This gap in knowledge has been an obstacle to new drug development.

The susceptibility to environmental irritants is likely to be determined by genetic factors. Knowing the genes associated with COPD susceptibility and development would be a significant step forward in better understanding the biology of COPD and identifying new drug targets. One such COPD-associated gene mutation has already been discovered; it is responsible for the COPD seen in patients with alpha-1 antitrypsin deficiency. Although this genetic defect is present in only a small number of patients with COPD, it has already paved the way for new therapeutic interventions and has served as a model for COPD in general.

How is it prevented, treated, and managed?

Prevention, treatment, staying healthy, prognosis

In the United States, the risk factor most strongly associated with COPD is cigarette smoking. Preventing teenagers from starting to smoke and getting established smokers to stop is clearly the most important way to prevent COPD. There are now many strategies to accomplish this, including public campaigns and personal counseling, higher costs for cigarettes, and new medications.

Another primary prevention strategy is to decrease occupational exposures to dusts, vapors, gases, and fumes. Treatment of asthma with disease modifying

Normal

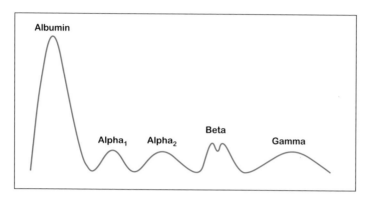

Alpha-1 antitrypsin deficiency

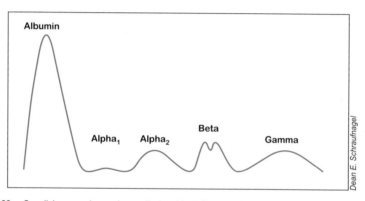

In 1963, a Swedish researcher and a medical resident discovered that the alpha-1 "clump" was missing in patients who developed emphysema at a young age. When they used electrophoresis, a method of purifying blood proteins, the absence of the alpha-1 protein became readily apparent.

anti-inflammatory agents to prevent airway remodeling may be another primary prevention strategy for COPD.

Secondary prevention aims to detect disease when it is still relatively mild and treatable. While there is evidence that this strategy works in cardiovascular disease and diabetes, evidence that the early detection and treatment of COPD improves outcomes is, at the moment, lacking, but it is an area of active investigation. The hope is that earlier intervention will improve the quality of life in these patients.

Tertiary prevention aims to lessen the complications of established disease. Treatment with bronchodilators, anti-inflammatory agents, and antibiotics according to guidelines can reduce exacerbations of the disease and prevent the accelerated decline in lung function (2). Reducing exposure to air pollution and getting influenza and pneumonia vaccines may also lessen the chance of exacerbations. Alpha-1 antitrypsin replacement is available for those with this deficiency. In advanced disease, oxygen therapy and pulmonary rehabilitation have been shown to be beneficial. In a small number of selected cases, lung surgery, including lung volume reduction surgery and lung transplantation, may be helpful.

At any stage of disease, avoidance of risk factors, such a tobacco smoke or occupational dusts, is important.

Are we making a difference?

Research past, present, and future

Important work by researchers in the 1950s and 1960s established that cigarette smoking was the major risk factor for disease in the developed world (6). The key intervention of decreasing smoking prevalence, which began with campaigns in the 1960s, has probably resulted in a lower prevalence of COPD compared to what might have been seen otherwise. However, over 20 percent of the U.S. adult population continues to smoke, and more people are exposed to second-hand smoke.

Recent investigations have demonstrated that asthma, ongoing inflammation in the lung, or the presence of other diseases may hasten the progression of COPD. Clinical trials suggest that medications may alter the natural history of disease.

Learning more about the basic biology of inflammation and how airways function is helping to develop new medications. A large National Institutes of Health research program called COPDGene (www.copdgene.org) is investigating the relationship between genetic and other risk factors and the development and progression of COPD. This project hopes to identify the genes involved in different aspects of COPD. This knowledge will then lead to a better understanding of how and why COPD develops. (For example, it appears that only about half of smokers will develop COPD.) These and other studies may help explain how COPD relates to other diseases of aging and frailty.

What we need to cure or eliminate COPD

Decreasing smoking prevalence in the population would, ultimately, reduce the prevalence of COPD. Current therapy is focused on improving the quality of life for patients, but more research on current tools, such as how to best intervene in early disease and when to use antibiotics, could make major differences. Combining epidemiology and basic biology to understand how and why exacerbations occur and what contributes to inflammation will be critically important. The genetic studies could lead to major breakthroughs. Of course, basic discoveries must be tested in clinical trials before their real benefit is known.

References

1. Mannino DM, Buist AS. Global burden of COPD: risk factors, prevalence, and future trends. *Lancet* 2007;370:765–773.
2. Celli BR, MacNee W. Standards for the diagnosis and treatment of patients with COPD: a summary of the ATS/ERS position paper. *Eur Respir J* 2004;23:932–946.
3. Mannino DM, Braman S. The epidemiology and economics of chronic obstructive pulmonary disease. *Proc Am Thorac Soc* 2007;4:502–506.
4. Centers for Disease Control and Prevention (CDC). Deaths from chronic obstructive pulmonary disease—United States, 2000–2005. *MMWR Morb Mortal Wkly Rep* 2008;57:1229–1232.
5. Chapman KR, Tashkin DP, Pye DJ. Gender bias in the diagnosis of COPD. *Chest* 2001;119:1691–1695.
6. Fletcher C, Peto R, Tinker CM, Speizer FE. The Natural History of Chronic Bronchitis and Emphysema. Oxford, UK: Oxford University Press; 1976.
7. Brown DW, Croft JB, Greenlund KJ, Giles WH. Trends in hospitalization with chronic obstructive pulmonary disease—United States, 1990–2005. *Am J Respir Crit Care Med* 2009;179:A4535.

Web sites of interest

American Lung Association
www.lungusa.org

National Heart, Lung, and Blood Institute
www.nhlbi.nih.gov/health/public/lung/copd/index.htm

Alpha-1 Foundation
www.alpha-1foundation.org

American Thoracic Society
http://patients.thoracic.org

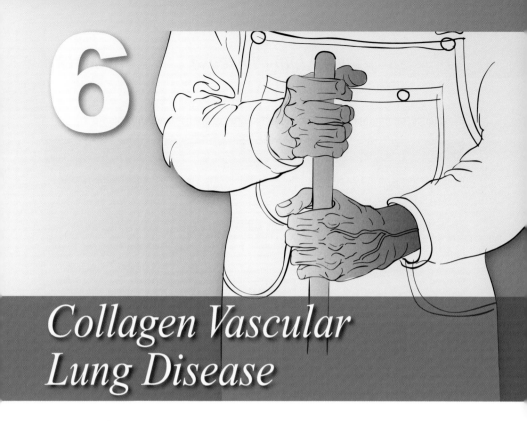

6

Collagen Vascular Lung Disease

Collagen vascular or connective tissue disorders are a group of autoimmune diseases in which antibodies attack the body's own organs and systems. Among the many targets of these auto-antibodies is connective tissue, which is the supporting structure for all of the body's cells.

An important component of connective tissue is the protein, collagen. Abnormalities in blood vessel structure and function are also typical, accounting for the term "collagen vascular diseases," which is often used interchangeably with connective tissue disorders. These disorders typically feature inflammation and scarring in several organs and tissues. The joints are frequently involved, particularly in the most common of these conditions, rheumatoid arthritis. Thus, rheumatology is the primary medical subspecialty involved in the diagnosis and care of these patients. Lung involvement may complicate the course of most of these conditions and sometimes can dominate the clinical picture.

Whom does it affect?

Epidemiology, prevalence, economic burden, and vulnerable populations

Some connective tissue disorders, notably rheumatoid arthritis and Sjögren's syndrome, are quite common, whereas scleroderma (systemic sclerosis) and

Prevalence, demographics, and common features of connective tissue disorders

Disorder	Prevalence	Demographics	Most frequent manifestations
Rheumatoid Arthritis	0.3–2.1 percent of population	Female to male ratio: 3 to 1; peak onset at age 35–50 years	Potentially disabling arthritis; increased risk of cardiovascular disease
Systemic Lupus Erythematosus (Lupus)	15–50/100,000	90% are females of child-bearing age; higher prevalence in African Americans	Fatigue, body aches, skin rash, neurologic complaints; effects on kidney, lung, heart
Scleroderma (Systemic Sclerosis)	19–75/100,000	Female to male ratio: 3:1; peak onset in 3rd–5th decades; more frequent in African Americans, Hispanics, and American Indians	Skin thickening; effects on vascular system, lung, kidney, gastrointestinal tract, heart
Sjögren's Syndrome	0.5–1 percent	Predominantly middle-aged women (female to male ratio: 9 to 1)	Dry eyes and dry mouth; effects on joints
Polymyositis	1/100,000	More common in women; all ages	Muscle weakness; difficulty swallowing; rash around eyes; effects on heart, lung

lupus (systemic lupus erythematosus) have an intermediate prevalence. All tend to strike mostly young and middle-aged women. They are more common in African Americans, in whom the severity of disease and, in particular, lung involvement is also higher. In the case of scleroderma, an especially vulnerable population is the Choctaw Native Americans in Oklahoma, in whom the prevalence is 469 per 100,000 (1).

The frequency and type of lung involvement in connective tissue disorders varies based on the underlying disease. Of all the connective tissue disorders, scleroderma is most likely to affect the lungs. Pulmonary fibrosis, also known as interstitial lung disease, which results in progressive scarring of the lungs, occurs in over two thirds of scleroderma patients (2). The most serious pulmonary complication of the connective tissue disorders is the involvement of the blood vessels in the lungs, which causes decreased oxygen uptake and pulmonary arterial hypertension (elevated blood pressure in the arteries of the lungs). This occurs in 10 to 15 percent of patients with scleroderma and in up to 5 percent of patients with the other conditions (2).

In lupus, pleurisy (inflammation of the lining around the lung) occurs in over one third of patients, often with pleural effusion (build-up of fluid around the lung) (3). Acute and potentially life-threatening types of lung involvement, such as alveolar hemorrhage (bleeding into the lung), are also observed in 5 to 15 percent of lupus patients (3). Evidence of narrowing of the bronchi on breathing tests is surprisingly common, observed in about one quarter of patients with rheumatoid arthritis and Sjögren's syndrome (4). Bronchiolitis (severe obstruction of the small airways) is an infrequent, but potentially devastating, complication of rheumatoid arthritis. Respiratory muscle weakness leading to shallow and difficult breathing can also occur in connective tissue disorders, especially polymyositis, which involves the muscles elsewhere in the body.

Lung infections are common in connective tissue disorders. This association may be related to the immunologic abnormalities accompanying the primary disease, aspiration of stomach or mouth contents into the lungs, or, most importantly, the effects of immunosuppressive agents used to treat these diseases. Recently, the advent of powerful new immunosuppresive agents (tumor necrosis factor blockers) for rheumatoid arthritis has placed renewed focus on the risks associated with immunosuppressant therapy. These agents may also increase the rates of tuberculosis and other serious infections (5). In lupus, up to half of all deaths are due to infections.

Connective tissue disorders exact a large economic burden on society. A common measure that integrates mortality and disability and can be thought of as a year of "healthy life" is Disability Adjusted Life Years (DALY). In a recent analysis, rheumatoid arthritis accounted for 98 DALY lost per 100,000 population in the United States, accounting for nearly 1 percent of all DALY lost (6). Direct healthcare costs have been estimated to be about $10,000 annually per patient (in 2006 dollars), plus a similar amount in lost productivity or indirect costs. Annual medical expenditures for lupus patients were over $12,000 (in 2005 dollars) per patient, greater than those for healthy control subjects; in patients with lupus and kidney involvement, costs were nearly four times greater than those for healthy control subjects (7). For scleroderma, a recent Canadian study estimated total annual costs (direct and indirect) at over $18,000 (2007 Canadian dollars; about $17,990 U.S. dollars) per patient (8). The relative contribution of lung involvement versus that of other organs to the overall economic burden, morbidity, and mortality of connective tissue disorders is variable and difficult to ascertain, but significant lung disease clearly has a substantial impact.

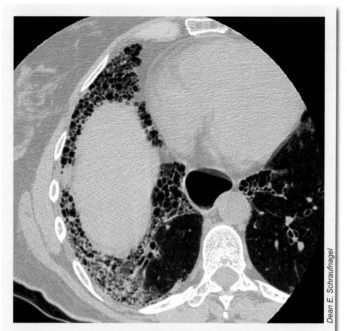

This computed tomography (CT) scan shows fibrosis and extensive regular cysts with a honeycomb-like appearance. The esophagus is also enlarged. Both of these features are often found in patients with scleroderma and lung involvement.

Dean E. Schraufnagel

What we are learning about the disease

Pathophysiology, causes: genetic, environment, microbes

The causes of connective tissue disorders are unknown, but intense research efforts are beginning to shed light on the mechanisms of tissue injury.

In rheumatoid arthritis, an infectious agent is suspected, but conclusive evidence has yet to emerge. Nonetheless, considerable progress has been made in delineating the cellular and molecular pathways involved in the joint and cartilage destruction of the disease, leading to the successful development of biologic agents that antagonize tumor necrosis factor, a key mediator of tissue damage.

In lupus, an interaction between susceptibility genes and environmental factors is believed to cause the disease. Hyperactivity of the immune system is a prominent feature, and variations in several genes that control the immune

Collagen Vascular Lung Disease

CASE STUDY

A 46-year-old Caucasian woman and mother of two children with a long-standing history of scleroderma was referred to a pulmonologist for activity-related shortness of breath occurring for the past year. Pulmonary fibrosis was noted on her chest radiograph, accompanied by a reduction in the lung capacity on pulmonary function tests. The scarring was treated with immunosuppressive medications for one year, and supplemental oxygen was started. Her symptoms and lung function tests improved, but 16 months later, her breathing became more labored, and she was hospitalized. An ultrasound of the heart (echocardiogram) demonstrated enlargement of the right side of the heart, with elevation on the estimated pulmonary artery pressure. Pulmonary hypertension was confirmed by right heart catheterization, and she was enrolled in a clinical research study of sildenafil, a drug that "relaxes" blood vessels and has been subsequently approved for treating pulmonary hypertension. With this treatment, she experienced a significant reduction in pulmonary artery pressure accompanied by an improvement in exercise capacity.

However, her condition gradually deteriorated with worsening pulmonary hypertension, despite the addition of a continuous intravenous medication, treprostinil. Lung transplantation was considered, but the procedure was considered too risky, given the extent of skin and esophageal disease. Her breathing continued to become more labored, with decreasing oxygen levels, until she died at age 50.

Comment

This case highlights the clinical challenges of lung involvement in scleroderma, which is the leading cause of death in this condition (2). Treatment options are limited and associated with potentially serious side effects. Moreover, the benefits of therapy are often small, and as this case illustrates, short-lived. Despite the availability of treatment, pulmonary hypertension associated with scleroderma carries a worse prognosis compared with other types of pulmonary hypertension, especially when accompanied by concomitant interstitial lung disease (9).

response increase the risk of lupus. The circulating auto-antibodies associated with lupus appear to be important in the disease process. They aggregate in specific tissues, induce inflammation and injury, and alter connective tissue cells. A similar inflammatory reaction is seen in Sjögren's syndrome and poly-myositis, targeting the salivary glands and muscles, respectively.

Injury to the endothelium (blood vessel cells) is believed to be the initiating pathologic event of scleroderma. This injury, perhaps mediated by immune cells or a viral infection, initiates a cascade of events resulting in narrowing of the small blood vessels, insufficient blood flow, and subsequent scarring. The fibrosis, or scarring, is marked by excessive and seemingly disorganized colla-gen deposition. Environmental exposures that have been associated with a small minority of cases of scleroderma include silica dust from coal and gold mining, polyvinyl chloride, epoxy resins, and aromatic hydrocarbons.

How is it prevented, treated, and managed?

Prevention, treatment, staying healthy, prognosis

Until its causes are positively established, there is no specific preventative strat-egy for the connective tissue disorders. However, smoking increases the risk of rheumatoid arthritis, and the disease is more severe in smokers, so smoking cessation is an important way to reduce the risk and severity of that disease.

The chronic inflammation in connective tissue disorders is associated with an increased risk of cardiovascular disease events, such as heart attack and stroke. In lupus, the risk of premature cardiovascular disease is increased up to 50-fold, and in rheumatoid arthritis, the risk of death due to a cardiovascular event is increased 50 percent compared with control subjects (10). In this respect, both lupus and rheumatoid arthritis are considered to be independent risk factors for cardiovascular disease, similar to hypertension, diabetes, and smoking. Thus, aggressive prevention of cardiovascular disease should be pur-sued. Strategies include maintaining a healthy diet, regular exercise, smoking cessation, and careful management of diabetes, high blood pressure, and high cholesterol. Statin drugs, which are used to lower cholesterol, may also have other benefits such as anti-oxidant and anti-inflammatory actions.

The treatment of connective tissue disorders depends on the specific disease, which organs are involved, and how rapidly the disease is progressing. Non-steroidal anti-inflammatory drugs (NSAIDs) are useful for pain, body aches, and fatigue. Anti-malarial drugs can reduce the skin and joint manifestations of lupus. Corticosteroids and other immunosuppressive drugs are useful to control inflam-mation and can be life-saving for patients with certain acute lung manifestations of lupus. The U.S. Food and Drug Administration (FDA) has approved several drugs for the treatment of pulmonary hypertension, which is often associated with connective tissue disorders. Unfortunately, scleroderma patients do not appear to benefit from these drugs as much as patients with other forms of pulmonary hypertension.

The prognosis of lung involvement in connective tissue disorders depends on the severity and type of underlying disease. Extensive lung disease, however, carries a 10-year survival rate of only 40 percent (2). The most serious chronic pulmonary manifestation of connective tissue disorders is pulmonary hypertension. Even with therapy, 3-year survival of pulmonary hypertension with scleroderma was only 47 percent in a recent large study from Britain (9).

Are we making a difference?

Research past, present, and future

Past research efforts have characterized the various clinical and pathologic features of respiratory involvement in the connective tissue diseases. With advances in molecular biology techniques, progress is now being made in characterizing the cellular and molecular pathways involved in tissue injury. In addition, associations with certain genetic variants involved in the immune response and the presence of specific auto-antibodies have been linked to these disorders.Understanding the mechanisms by which the different lung manifestations occur and the variations that patients have should identify which molecules are involved in the disease and allow new therapeutic targets to be developed. For example, why do some patients with scleroderma experience no or minimal lung disease, some develop severe interstitial lung disease or pulmonary hypertension, and some develop both?

Large, well-designed clinical trials will continue to be fundamental for bringing new, safe, and effective treatments to clinical practice. The relatively low prevalence of lung disease in connective tissue disorders other than scleroderma makes such trials challenging. Success has been achieved in scleroderma, where a multi-institutional network, the Scleroderma Lung Study, is testing therapies for interstitial lung disease (11). In pulmonary hypertension, after an initial early trial restricted to scleroderma patients (12), subsequent study designs have incorporated connective tissue disorders as a subset within a larger group of subjects without connective tissue disorders. Although this approach has facilitated the approval of

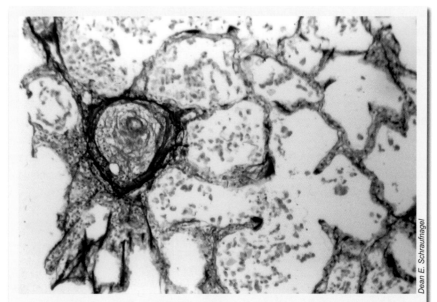

This small pulmonary artery is constricted by the growth and layering of the inside cells to greatly hinder blood flow, a feature of scleroderma.

novel agents for these patients, it does not allow us to understand fully the role of these drugs in pulmonary hypertension associated with connective tissue disorders, which may be different from other forms of pulmonary hypertension.

What we need to cure or eliminate collagen vascular lung disease

The collagen vascular diseases are almost certainly multi-factorial in origin, and thus, it is unlikely that a single "magic bullet" will be discovered to cure all of them. Continued study of the highly complex immune system and how the body turns against itself in the process of autoimmunity, however, will likely indentify key molecules involved in these processes. The next steps would be to identify ways to bypass or correct the defects and to understand how these factors interact with environmental factors to trigger the diseases and their pulmonary complications. Close collaboration between clinicians and basic scientists will be critical to the success of such efforts. A most important element will be the patients themselves who will take the time and make the effort to participate in the clinical research studies needed to find a cure.

References

1. Mayes MD. Scleroderma epidemiology. *Rheum Dis Clin North Am* 2003;29:239–254.
2. Wells AU, Steen V, Valentini G. Pulmonary complications: one of the most challenging complications of systemic sclerosis. *Rheumatology (Oxford)* 2009;48(suppl 3):iii40–iii44.
3. Memet B, Ginzler EM. Pulmonary manifestations of systemic lupus erythematosus. *Semin Respir Crit Care Med* 2007;28:441–450.
4. Gauhar UA, Gaffo AL, Alarcón GS. Pulmonary manifestations of rheumatoid arthritis. *Semin Respir Crit Care Med* 2007;28:430–440.
5. Patkar NM, Teng GG, Curtis JR, Saag KG. Association of infections and tuberculosis with antitumor necrosis factor alpha therapy. *Curr Opin Rheumatol* 2008;20:320–326.
6. Lundkvist J, Kastäng F, Kobelt G. The burden of rheumatoid arthritis and access to treatment: health burden and costs. *Eur J Health Econ* 2008;8(suppl 2):S49–S60.
7. Carls G, Li T, Panopalis P, Wang S, Mell AG, Gibson TB, Goetzel RZ. Direct and indirect costs to employers of patients with systemic lupus erythematosus with and without nephritis. *J Occup Environ Med* 2009;51:66–79.
8. Bernatsky S, Hudson M, Panopalis P, Clarke AE, Pope J, Leclercq S, St Pierre Y, Baron M. The cost of systemic sclerosis. *Arthritis Rheum* 2009;61:119–123.
9. Condliffe R, Kiely DG, Peacock AJ, Corris PA, Gibbs JS, Vrapi F, Das C, Elliot CA, Johnson M, DeSoyza J, *et al*. Connective tissue disease-associated pulmonary arterial hypertension in the modern treatment era. *Am J Respir Crit Care Med* 2009;179:151–157.
10. Kaplan MJ. Management of cardiovascular disease risk in chronic inflammatory disorders. *Nat Rev Rheumatol* 2009;5:208–217.
11. Tashkin DP, Elashoff R, Clements PJ, Goldin J, Roth MD, Furst DE, Arriola E, Silver R, Strange C, Bolster M, *et al*. Cyclophosphamide versus placebo in scleroderma lung disease. *N Engl J Med* 2006; 354:2655–2666.
12. Badesch DB, Tapson VF, McGoon MD, Brundage BH, Rubin LJ, Wigley FM, Rich S, Barst RJ, Barrett PS, Kral KM, *et al*. Continuous intravenous epoprostenol for pulmonary hypertension due to the scleroderma spectrum of disease. A randomized, controlled trial. *Ann Intern Med* 2000;132:425–434.

Web sites of interest

Arthritis Foundation
www.arthritis.org

Lupus Foundation of America
www.lupus.org

Scleroderma Foundation
www.scleroderma.org

Pulmonary Hypertension Association
www.phassociation.org

Coalition for Pulmonary Fibrosis
www.coalitionforpf.org

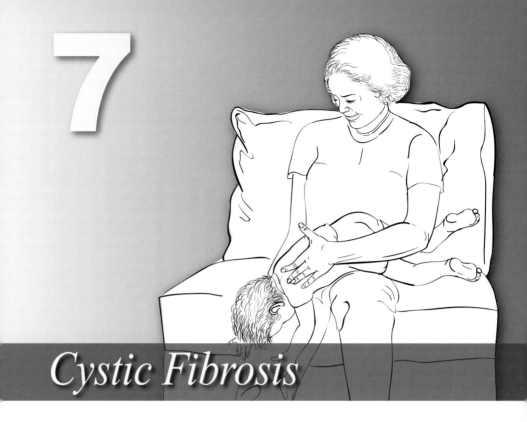

7

Cystic Fibrosis

Cystic fibrosis (CF) is the most common, life-shortening genetic disease in Caucasians. It affects the transport of salt and water across cells and affects different organs, but lung disease is responsible for the majority of symptoms, burden of care, and lost years of life. The gene that causes the disease has now been identified and sequenced.

Whom does it affect?

Epidemiology, prevalence, economic burden, vulnerable populations

Cystic fibrosis affects at least 30,000 people in the United States; between 900 and 1,000 new cases are diagnosed every year (1). One in 29 people of Caucasian ancestry is an unaffected carrier of the CF gene mutation. In the United States, cystic fibrosis occurs at a rate of 1 in 3,400 births. While it occurs in persons of all racial and ethnic backgrounds, it is most common in Caucasians of Northern European ancestry. Historically, half of affected individuals were diagnosed by five months of age, though the average age at diagnosis was five years, and some individuals were not diagnosed until adulthood.

Median predicted survival age for those born with cystic fibrosis

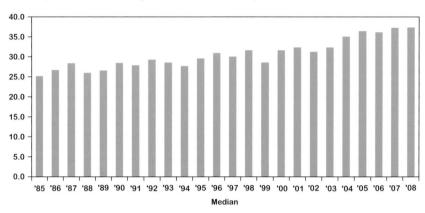

Median

Those with cystic fibrosis are living longer thanks to a number of factors, including chest physiotherapy and better antibiotics, nutrition, and overall care. Cystic Fibrosis Foundation Web site. *Cystic Fibrosis Patient Registry: Annual Data Report 2008.* Available at: http://www.cff.org/LivingWithCF/Quality Improvement/PatientRegistryReport. Accessed March 20, 2010.

In 2010, however, all states began requiring that newborns undergo screening for cystic fibrosis. This should be helpful because early diagnosis and treatment reduce symptoms, improve health, and reduce costs associated with disease complications.

When CF was first described, most affected children died in infancy or early childhood. With improvements in nutritional therapy, antibiotics, and chest physiotherapy, life was extended into the second decade, and with continued attention to improving care, median survival has increased to 37.4 years, according to the most recent Cystic Fibrosis Foundation registry data. Today, about half of all patients are adults, and although the quality of life is lower than that of the general population, it has been steadily improving.

The cost of treating cystic fibrosis is very high. Most affected individuals must take pancreatic enzymes to digest food effectively, and some require insulin for diabetes mellitus. Many drugs that prevent and treat pulmonary complications are expensive. The average cost of care for a person with CF living in the United States in 2006 was just over $48,000, more than 20 times higher than that for someone without CF (2). Medications account for the single highest expenditure, followed by hospitalization. Each year, one in three patients with CF is hospitalized, mostly for treatment of "pulmonary exacerbations" caused by an infection requiring intravenous antibiotics. Time lost from work and school is

CASE STUDY

A male child was born in 1980. He did not gain weight normally and had frequent, loose, foul-smelling bowel movements. At four months of age, he developed a cough that produced phlegm. A sweat test showed elevated chloride levels, which are diagnostic of cystic fibrosis. He was referred to a CF center and was treated with pancreatic enzymes, chest physiotherapy (to clear excessive secretions in the chest), and antibiotics. He was in fairly good health for a number of years, although he struggled to gain weight and had several hospital stays for breathing problems. At age 10, he became infected with the bacterium Pseudomonas aeruginosa. *His pulmonary function worsened, and he required hospital stays lasting up to two weeks once or twice a year. At age 14, he began taking a new drug, dornase alfa, and showed improvement. Three years later, he began taking nebulized tobramycin, and showed further improvement. When he turned 18, he transitioned to an adult CF program. He continued to have frequent pulmonary exacerbations requiring repeated courses of intravenous antibiotics. He developed complications from the antibiotics, including kidney damage and hearing loss. At age 24, he received a lung transplant. He now maintains normal lung function but takes several medications to prevent infection and lung rejection. He works part time and takes classes at a community college.*

Comment

This case is representative of an early presentation of an infant with cystic fibrosis with malabsorption and failure to thrive symptoms. Going forward, most patients will be diagnosed by newborn screening, which is now mandatory in all states. He developed bronchiectasis at an early age and became infected with the bacterium Pseudomonas aeruginosa, *the most important infection for CF patients. He had severe pulmonary disease as marked by frequent pulmonary exacerbations, rapid loss of lung function, and need for a lung transplant.*

common in CF. If indirect costs such as these are factored in, the overall expense is significantly higher. In addition to the cost, the treatment burden for CF patients is also significant. On average, CF patients spend nearly two hours a day performing therapies in order to maintain their health. For young children, this imposes a substantial burden on the family.

What we are learning about this disease

Pathophysiology, causes: genetic, environment, microbes

Cystic fibrosis was referred to in medieval folklore, which mentions infants with salty skin who were considered "bewitched" because they routinely died an early death. Salty skin is now recognized as a sign of CF. It was not until 1936, however, that Dr. Guido Fanconi named this condition "cystic fibrosis with bronchiectasis." In 1949, Dr. Charles Upton Lowe established that CF was a genetic disorder, and in 1953, Dr. Paul A. di Sant'Agnese reported that children with CF secrete excessive salt in their sweat after observing dehydration in these children during a New York City heat wave. This finding is the basis of the "sweat test," used to diagnose cystic fibrosis (3).

Much of research until the 1990s was aimed at learning more about the physiology of the surface layer of cells and why salt transport in tissues was defective. After discovering how to unravel the genetic code, the focus and tempo of research switched. In 1989, a collaborative effort using new molecular techniques led to the discovery of the genetic abnormality that causes CF and the sequencing of this gene. Cystic fibrosis is caused by mutations in the cystic fibrosis transmembrane regulator (CFTR) gene. A recessive genetic disorder, it is inherited when two carrier parents (who have one normal gene and one gene with a mutation) each contributes the abnormal CFTR gene to their child. Thus, the likelihood that two carrier parents will have an affected child is 1:4 for *each* pregnancy. Carriers do not usually have symptoms of CF, but carrier status can be detected through genetic testing.

The abnormality in the CFTR gene causes a defective CFTR protein to be produced, resulting in abnormal transport of salt (sodium and chloride) and water across cells that line the respiratory, digestive, and genital tracts. This results in a reduction of water in the fluid lining the airways. Diminished water causes the respiratory secretions to become thicker and clog small airways. The stagnant sputum becomes infected as bacteria that are inhaled or brought into the lungs through the mouth become lodged there. Persistent stagnation allows persistent infection and chronic inflammation to develop. Inflammatory cells trapped in the sputum add to its tenacity. *Pseudomonas aeruginosa* and other bacteria from the environment thrive in the mucus that is retained in the airways of the CF lung. The bronchi dilate and their walls weaken, setting up a condition called bronchiectasis that results in further airflow obstruction. The vicious cycle of airway

Cystic Fibrosis

obstruction, inflammation, and persistent infection leads to a progressive decline in lung function and eventually causes respiratory failure and death.

Clogged mucus secretions in the digestive tract can lead to malnutrition and vitamin deficiencies. The genital tract abnormality can lead to infertility in men and women. Other complications include CF-related diabetes, liver cirrhosis, bowel obstruction, chronic sinusitis, and osteoporosis. There is a high prevalence of depression and anxiety in CF patients.

Environmental exposures worsen CF lung disease. Children who are exposed to tobacco smoke have lower lung function and more pulmonary exacerbations than those who live in smoke-free environments. High levels of air pollution are associated with an increased rate of adverse pulmonary events.

How is it prevented, treated, and managed?

Prevention, treatment, staying healthy, prognosis

Cystic fibrosis carrier testing is recommended for Caucasian women who are considering pregnancy or who are pregnant. This can allow a couple who is at risk of having a child with CF to use reproductive technologies to avoid having a baby with CF, or to prepare for the birth of an infant with CF. Diagnosing CF before a child is born, or by newborn screening, allows earlier referral to a CF center and initiation of treatment with pancreatic enzymes before symptoms of abnormal absorption or poor growth occur.

In the United States, most people with CF are treated at specialized CF centers accredited by the Cystic Fibrosis Foundation. Multidisciplinary teams of physicians, nurses, respiratory therapists, dietitians, and social workers care for both adult and pediatric patients.

Individuals with CF who have better nutrition have higher lung function and longer life expectancy. Nutritional management with pancreatic enzymes and a high-calorie, liberal-fat diet is recommended from the time of diagnosis. Some people with CF benefit from supplemental feedings given overnight by a tube placed into the stomach. Specialized vitamin preparations are prescribed in order to reduce the risk of deficiency of certain fat-soluble vitamins.

Although most infants and young children have only intermittent symptoms of cough and wheezing, recent research shows that there are structural and functional abnormalities of the lung as early as the first few months of life. Most CF treatments for lung disease have been tested primarily in patients aged five and older. These treatments include physical methods to clear thick secretions from the chest, the use of hand-held devices that cause an oscillation in the airways during expiration, and vests that provide external oscillations to the chest wall. Maintenance medications include those that thin sticky airway secretions, such as dornase alfa and hypertonic saline, bronchodilators such as albuterol, inhaled antibiotics such as tobramycin, and anti-inflammatory drugs such as ibuprofen and azithromycin. Practice guidelines assist physicians and patients in choosing appropriate therapies (4).

Frequent monitoring of nutrition and pulmonary function and screening for complications of CF are essential components of care. Current recommendations include quarterly visits to an accredited CF center, frequent pulmonary function testing and respiratory cultures, and annual screening tests for complications, including liver disease and diabetes. Prompt treatment of lung infections and worsening symptoms is extremely important.

Are we making a difference?

Research past, present, and future

Better understanding of the disease and application of this understanding are responsible for the steadily improving life expectancy in persons with CF. Prevention and treatment of respiratory infections may reduce the vicious cycle of bronchiectasis. Prevention of chronic *Pseudomonas aeruginosa* infection is now a goal of therapy for infants and young children. This strategy consists of frequent monitoring with sputum cultures and treatment with appropriate antibiotics whenever *P. aeruginosa* is found. Vaccines intended to prevent *P. aeruginosa* infection and new antibiotics to treat it are being developed.

Many new drugs that may help people affected with CF are being studied. Investigational drugs that help improve salt transport across cells include denufosol, which activates a non-CFTR chloride channel to increase the volume of airway surface liquid. Other potential treatments for infections are also being studied.

Among the most exciting advances in drug therapies for CF are new drugs that have been designed to correct the basic defect in the CFTR protein. The development and early clinical studies of these drugs have been complex, as different gene mutations cause different problems in protein production; therefore, these drugs are specific to defined gene mutations. Some of these drugs

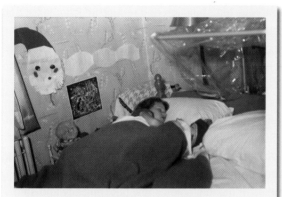

As a young girl, Joan Finnegan Brooks was "allowed" by her parents to sleep outside of her mist tent on Christmas Eve. Mist tents are no longer used because other therapies have proven more effective, and the tents increased the risk of bacterial infections in the child's lungs.

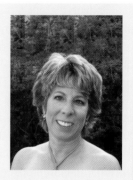

At age 50, Ms. Finnegan Brooks embodies the advances in cystic fibrosis management that have greatly extended the lives of people with this disease.

have been shown to improve CFTR function as measured by improved sweat chloride levels and nasal potential differences, a way of directly measuring salt transport across the nasal membranes.

Survival has more than doubled over the last 40 years in conjunction with a greater understanding of the basic pathophysiology in CF. Because a single aberrant gene and its protein product are now known, research can concentrate on measures to correct this defect. If this research leads to another doubling of the lifespan in the next 40 years, life expectancy would approach normal. Application of these findings, however, would only be a part of the effort. Continued attention and research on the management of the patients will be needed to optimize not only length of life, but quality of life, for people living with cystic fibrosis.

What we need to cure or eliminate cystic fibrosis

The implementation of newborn screening for CF in every state will facilitate earlier diagnosis and initiation of therapies to preserve good nutrition and lung function. This may translate into better lung function over the long term and improved survival.

Though therapies that improve lung function and reduce infection exist and are a mainstay of therapy, more therapies with alternative mechanisms of action are needed. Therapies designed to improve chloride secretion in the airways or increase hydration of airway mucus may improve bronchial hygiene and preserve lung function. This could translate into improved survival.

While gene therapy has not yet lived up to its initial promise, research is ongoing to develop a safe, efficient method for delivering a normal CFTR gene to the airways of CF patients. Successful gene therapy could lead to a cure for CF.

Drugs designed to improve the function of mutant CFTR, thus correcting the ion transport problem, are currently in development. Several such drugs are in Phase 2 and Phase 3 studies. If these studies show both efficacy and safety, these drugs may lead to stabilization or improvement of CF lung disease and allow for prolonged survival.

References

1. O'Sullivan BP, Freedman SD. Cystic fibrosis. *Lancet* 2009;373:1891–1904.
2. Ouyang L, Grosse SD, Amendah DD, Schechter MS. Healthcare expenditures for privately insured people with cystic fibrosis. *Pediatr Pulmonol* 2009;44:989–996.
3. Farrell PM, Rosenstein BJ, White TB, Accurso FJ, Castellani C, Cutting GR, Durie PR, Legrys VA, Massie J, Parad RB et al. Guildeines for diagnosis of cystic fibrosis in newborns through older adults: Cystic Fibrosis Foundation consensus report. *J Pediatr* 2008; 153: S4-S14.
4. Flume PA, O'Sullivan BP, Robinson KA, Goss CH, Mogayzel PJ Jr, Willey-Courand DB, Bujan J, Finder J, Lester M, Quittell L, *et al.* Cystic fibrosis pulmonary guidelines: chronic medications for maintenance of lung health. *Am J Respir Crit Care Med* 2007;176:957–969.

Web sites of interest

Cystic Fibrosis Foundation
www.cff.org

Cystic Fibrosis Research, Inc.
www.cfri.org

United States Adult Cystic Fibrosis Association
www.usacfa.org

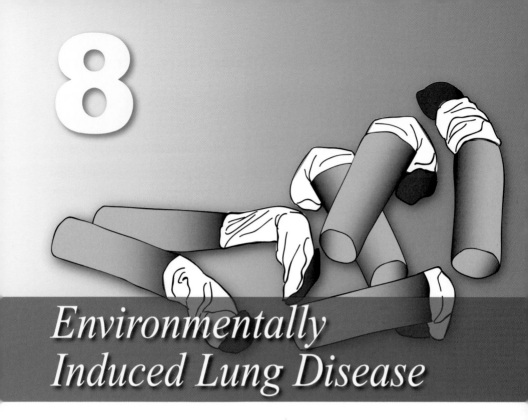

8

Environmentally Induced Lung Disease

Many environmental factors contribute to the development of respiratory diseases. The World Health Organization's 2002 report "Reducing Risks, Promoting Healthy Life" emphasized the importance of environmental factors in lung disease and stated that controlling air pollution and tobacco consumption would be among the most important interventions to promote good health (1). The report noted that the burden of lung disease is unevenly distributed and can be traced to regional environmental challenges, nutrition, and poverty, as well as to a person's underlying state of health. Because of the difficulty in assessing the prevalence and amount of exposure, the precise risk each environment poses is unknown. Risk assessment is further complicated by socioeconomic and genetic factors that may predispose a person to respiratory disease or alter the prognosis. However, by understanding the mechanisms of disease, defining high-risk populations, and intervening to mitigate or reduce environmental exposures, the burden of disease may be significantly lessened.

Whom does it affect?

Epidemiology, prevalence, economic burden, vulnerable populations

The lungs are the main interface between the body and the environment. Consequently, the lungs are a common site of environmentally induced disease. Thousands of environmental toxins and commercial chemicals are now in use, the particles of which may become aerosolized or airborne in the form of fibers, fumes, mists, or dust. Inhabitants of major metropolitan areas may inhale more than 2 milligrams of dust each day, and workers in dusty occupations may inhale up to 100 times that amount.

The lungs are equipped with a complex system to reduce the effect of potentially harmful inhaled toxins and to preserve the sensitive gas exchange mechanism of the alveolar surface, so pulmonary function in most persons is rarely affected despite this exposure. Nevertheless, environmentally related lung disease has increased over the past several decades, probably owing to exposure to respiratory toxins, mainly tobacco smoke and air pollutants.

Understanding and quantifying the contributions of environmental exposures to lung disease is difficult because individuals respond differently to the same factors. The variations in response arise from different susceptibilities,

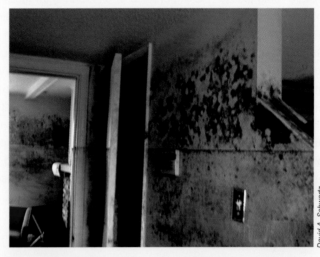

Water damage can cause mold to grow on walls. The mold can stimulate hypersensitivity pneumonitis or an asthma-like illness.

David A. Schwartz

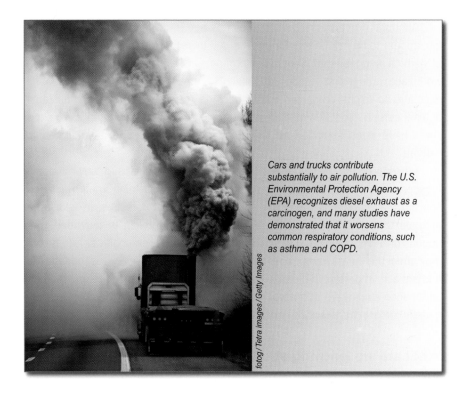

Cars and trucks contribute substantially to air pollution. The U.S. Environmental Protection Agency (EPA) recognizes diesel exhaust as a carcinogen, and many studies have demonstrated that it worsens common respiratory conditions, such as asthma and COPD.

fotog / Tetra images / Getty Images

including genetic predisposition, developmental stages of life, presence of co-existing diseases, other exposures, and lifestyle differences such as varying nutritional status and physical activity levels. Despite the difficulties inherent in teasing apart environmental contributions to human disease, a number of studies have shown that environmental exposures, particularly during fetal development, can profoundly affect subsequent genetic expression.

For example, environmental factors are known to play important roles in the pathogenesis of asthma—both in terms of main effects and those exerted indirectly through complex interactions with gene variants. The increase in the prevalence, incidence, and severity of asthma over the last 20 years, along with epidemiologic studies on the environment, provides strong evidence that exposures, including air pollution, play an important role in the development of this disease. These changes have occurred too rapidly to be accounted for by genetic changes in the population.

Although demographic factors, such as age, race, and socioeconomic status, appear to be risk factors for asthma, the increasing prevalence and severity of asthma suggest that airborne allergens, smoking behavior, agents in the workplace, indoor and outdoor air pollution, viruses, domestic and occupational exposure to toxins contained within bacteria (endotoxins), and immunization against certain infectious diseases play a role as well. Moreover, *in utero* exposures have been identified as important risk factors for the development of asthma.

While prenatal exposure to diesel exhaust particles and environmental tobacco smoke is associated with an increased risk of asthma, maternal ingestion of fruits, vegetables, and oily fish appears to be protective. In addition, it appears that gestational exposure to an environment rich in microbial compounds protects against the development of allergic hypersensitivity (atopy) and may affect the innate immune response to allergens. However, host genetic factors are also important in disease development; people exposed to environmental tobacco smoke are at greater risk of developing asthma if they carry certain genetic factors (for example, those found at chromosome 17q21).

What are we learning about this disease?

Pathophysiology, causes: genetic, environment, microbes

The development of environmentally induced lung disease is a function of the toxicity of the inhaled substance, the intensity and duration of exposure, and an individual's susceptibility. The physical state of the inhaled substance (for example, solid, fume, or mixture), the size, and other characteristics (for example, solubility) principally determine the initial site of disease activity. Smaller particles (0.1 to 1.0 microns) are more likely to reach the lungs' alveoli, but airborne particles up to 5 microns in size may also do so. In general, larger particles (10 microns or greater) are trapped and removed by the mucus and cilia of the upper respiratory tract.

Although the respiratory tract is quite resilient in the face of the plethora of agents in the environment, disruption of mechanisms to clear inhaled material may occur if an individual is exposed to highly concentrated particles in certain situations or if an exposure occurs during strenuous labor. Depending on the inhaled substance, acute or chronic reactions occur as particles are deposited on the alveolar surface. Acute reactions are characterized by swelling (edema) and inflammation,

CASE STUDY

A 55-year-old woman sought medical attention for progressive breathlessness. She grew up in a household where her father smoked. She herself smoked on average a pack of cigarettes per day for 40 years and worked with rosin solder. Five years earlier, she had developed breathlessness, and two years earlier she had to stop working because of this symptom. Since then, her condition worsened, and she required 2 liters of supplemental oxygen per minute. She remembered that working with solder increased her shortness of breath, as did days with high air pollution. She used a wood stove in winter for heat and had a cat in the home, to which she was allergic. Her father died of emphysema.

A pulmonologist found wheezes with prolonged expiration. Her pulmonary function tests showed severe obstruction (which improved after she inhaled a bronchodilator), trapped air in her lungs, and markedly reduced diffusing capacity—a measure of oxygen transfer through the lungs. She was continued on oxygen and inhalers, and given advice and help to quit smoking. She was advised to remove the cat from her home, stop using the wood stove, and stay indoors on high air pollution days.

Comment

This case depicts the complexity of assessing the impact that various environmental factors may have on the cause or aggravation of lung disease. In what appears to be well-defined respiratory disease of a known cause, such as chronic obstructive pulmonary disease (COPD) due to tobacco use, many other environmental factors may contribute to the onset of disease and worsening of symptoms with disease progression.

Most lung diseases are considered to be of unknown cause (idiopathic) unless there are strong clinical, physiologic, and pathologic associations with an environmental etiology. Of note, environmental factors can result in most types of lung disease, including asthma, COPD, interstitial lung disease, infectious lung disease, pulmonary hypertension, and lung cancer. These and other lung diseases, including genetically determined diseases such as cystic fibrosis and alpha-1 antitrypsin deficiency, may be aggravated by environmental factors. Unless environmental factors are considered, an important opportunity for case finding, treatment, and prevention of future disease will be missed.

Number of sites above National Ambient Air Quality Standards

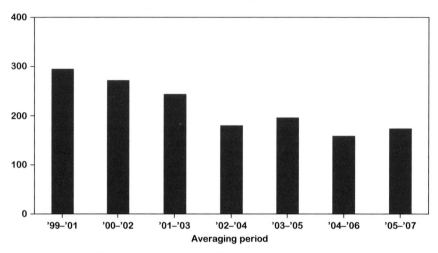

This graph shows that the number of sites, out of 728 tested, exceeding the air quality standards for particulate matter (soot) in the United States has decreased over time. Nevertheless, approximately 1 in 4 sites monitored still exceeds national standards. U.S. Environmental Protection Agency Web site. Available at: http://www.epa.gov/airtrends/pm.html. Accessed March 20, 2010.

while chronic reactions are characterized by connective tissue scarring (fibrosis) and the formation of specific aggregates of immune cells (granulomas).

Several factors may make certain individuals more susceptible to inhaled toxins. These include genetic tendencies, the inability to clear substances from the lower respiratory tract, the presence of coexisting pulmonary diseases, and the effects of concomitant exposures, such as cigarette smoke.

Environmental lung diseases are difficult to diagnose and study epidemiologically because of the extended time from exposure to clinical expression of disease, which often ranges from years to decades. In addition, individuals can be exposed to several substances at one time, and they may work in a number of professions and do a variety of tasks in their lifetime (2–4).

How is it prevented, treated, and managed?

Prevention, treatment, staying healthy, prognosis

The first step in preventing environmentally related lung disease is to recognize the exposure–disease relationship. Then, primary prevention is achieved with reduction, modification, or elimination of the exposure or environment. These changes may involve behavior modifications at the individual level, such as smoking cessation. Other interventions require societal and global approaches to prioritize and target environmental modifications with public health policy implications. Some of these efforts necessitate legislation and public policy for implementation, such as the use of air quality standards to reduce air pollution or bans on the advertisement of tobacco products or on smoking in public places to reduce tobacco smoke. Education is an important aspect of prevention of environmentally induced lung disease.

The treatment of environmentally induced lung disease usually includes recommendations for exposure reduction or modification to reduce disease

Annual prevalence of smoking

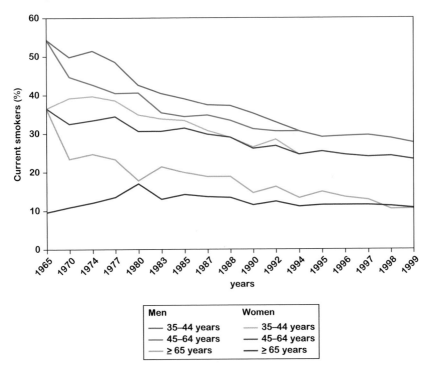

The number of Americans who smoke has declined steadily from 1965 to 1999. The decline is most dramatic among men, but rates have declined among women as well, except among those age 65 or older. National Center for Health Statistics.

impairment. The prognosis of environmentally induced lung diseases is usually dictated by the underlying disease and not always by the environment itself, except in some occupational lung diseases. However, it is important to remember that, as a group, these are preventable diseases.

Are we making a difference?

Research past, present, and future

Significant strides have been made in linking environmental factors and lung disease by using epidemiologic and toxicologic studies combined with an effort to determine the mechanisms by which the disease develops. This approach has resulted in a reduction in occupational lung disease caused by dust, called *pneumoconiosis*, and asbestos-related lung disease in communities surrounding industrial sources. In addition, the ongoing recognition of new environmental factors in lung disease, such as exposure to smoke from burning wood and other plants commonly used in developing countries for heat, has been an important accomplishment in this area.

What we need to cure or eliminate environmentally induced lung disease

The cornerstone of controlling, reducing, and eliminating environmentally associated respiratory disease is improving indoor, outdoor, and workplace air quality in the United States. In addition, several important advances are necessary (5). First, the ability to assess the environment and the exposure must be improved in order to understand the impact environmental factors have on disease and to determine whether new environmental factors might result in disease. Assessment methods are needed that can monitor a person's total exposure to environmental factors over a lifetime instead of during a certain time period or in one situation. This assessment could be accomplished at least partially with the development of biomarkers that indicate exposure to precipitating factors from *in utero* to the end of life. Research efforts that address the complexity of the exposures are most likely to show the effect of environmental factors on lung disease.

Second, more needs to be learned about the interaction between the individual and the environment to better define at-risk populations. These efforts

Average serum cotinine levels (nanograms per milliliter) of nonsmokers

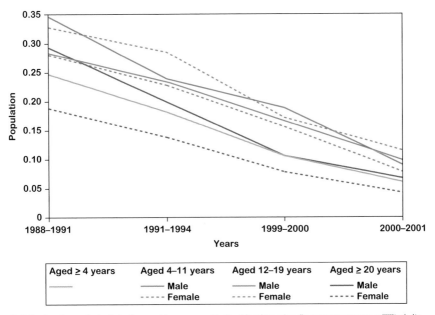

Cotinine is a byproduct of nicotine and is measured in the blood or urine (in nanograms per milliliter). Its presence in nonsmokers indicates their level of tobacco smoke exposure and risk for disease caused by secondhand smoke. National Health and Nutrition Examination Survey.

should not only identify populations at high risk for disease but should also consider how modifications of environmental factors could reduce disease impact. An integrative approach will be required for these research efforts, including reliance on advancing genetic technologies, along with bioinformatics and complex biostatistical methodologies. In addition to identifying genetic factors associated with risk of exposure, this research could identify biomarkers of disease and define potential pathogenic pathways that may be targeted to reduce or treat disease.

Third, the mechanisms by which environmental toxins affect disease development need to be defined. Although it is well-established that outdoor air pollution increases the risk of cardiovascular disease and indoor air pollution due to biomass smoke increases risk of childhood infection, the molecular pathways by which these toxicants exert their effect are unknown.

Finally, to control environmental lung disease on a population basis, multi-disciplinary research and public health programs are needed to translate what is learned about these toxins and molecular pathways into environmental change to help people who are at risk of respiratory disease. At present, there are too few researchers and clinicians who have an interest and ability to conduct environmental research. Thus, an important first step to move this field forward is to train more researchers. With these approaches and the development of partnerships between researchers and the public at large, the role of environmental factors in lung disease will continue to be defined and methods to prevent disease will be implemented.

References

1. World Health Organization. *The World Health Report 2002—Reducing Risks, Promoting Healthy Life.* Available at: http://www.who.int/whr/2002/en. Accessed February 20, 2010.
2. Centers for Disease Control and Prevention. *2006 Surgeon General's Report—The Health Consequences of Involuntary Exposure to Tobacco Smoke.* Available at: http://www.cdc.gov/tobacco/data_statistics/sgr/2006/index.htm. Accessed February 20, 2010.
3. United States Environmental Protection Agency. Learn the issues. Available at: http://www.epa.gov/epahome/learn.htm. Accessed February 20, 2010.
4. National Institutes of Environmental Health Sciences—National Institutes of Health. Environmental health topics: conditions & diseases. Available at: http://www.niehs.nih.gov/health/topics/index.cfm. Accessed February 20, 2010.
5. Crapo JD, Broaddus VC, Brody AR, Malindzak G, Samet J, Wright JR for the American Thoracic Society. Workshop on lung disease and the environment: where do we go from here? *Am J Respir Crit Care Med* 2003;168:250–254.

Web sites of interest

World Health Organization
The World Health Report 2002—Reducing Risks, Promoting Healthy Life
www.who.int/whr/2002/en/

Centers for Disease Control and Prevention
2006 Surgeon General's Report—The Health Consequences of Involuntary Exposure to Tobacco Smoke
www.cdc.gov/tobacco/data_statistics/sgr/2006/index.htm

United States Environmental Protection Agency
Learn the Issues
www.epa.gov/epahome/learn.htm

National Institute of Environmental Health Science—National Institutes of Health Environmental Health Topics: Conditions & Diseases
www.niehs.nih.gov/health/topics/index.cfm

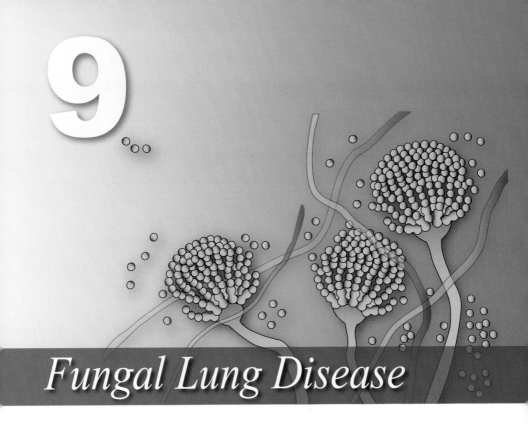

9

Fungal Lung Disease

Fungal infections of the lung are less common than bacterial and viral infections but pose significant problems in diagnosis and treatment. They mainly affect people living in certain geographic areas and those with immune deficiency. Their virulence varies from causing no symptoms to causing death.

Whom does it affect?

Epidemiology, prevalence, economic burden, vulnerable populations

Rates of invasive fungal infections have surged during recent decades, largely because of the increasing size of the population at risk. This population includes patients who are immunosuppressed because of diseases, such as cancers of immune cells of the blood, bone marrow, and lymph nodes, and those with human immunodeficiency virus (HIV) infection. It also includes patients taking immunosuppressive drugs, which are given to avoid rejection of transplanted organs or stem cells and as treatment for autoimmune diseases, such as rheumatoid arthritis. Immunosuppressive drugs are also given to reduce inflammation. For example, corticosteroids are often prescribed for many different lung diseases. A new class of potent immunosuppressive agents includes compounds that block regulatory molecules produced by the immune system called cytokines.

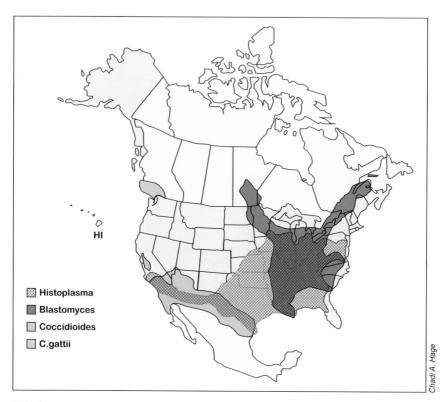

Histoplasmosis occurs primarily in the areas of the Ohio and Mississippi rivers. Blastomycosis occurs in the central and southeastern United States. Coccidioidomycosis is limited to the southwestern United States. Infection with Cryptococcus gattii *occurs in the northwestern United States. The area of histoplasmin skin test positivity in the southwestern United States probably represents cross-reactivity caused by coccidioidomycosis.*

One of these cytokines, tumor necrosis factor, is key to many of the body's immune processes. In addition, patients with chronic debilitating diseases, who are in an immune-deficient state, make an attractive host for invasive fungi.

Massive population growth, urban development, and climate change are also factors that have increased the prevalence of fungal infections in certain areas and are putting more people at risk of becoming infected with the fungi that is endemic to where they live. More recently, natural disasters such as tsunamis and hurricanes have also contributed to the changing epidemiology of fungal infections.

The financial and social burdens of fungal infections are staggering. Using National Hospital Discharge Data Sets from 1998, the annual cost of fungal

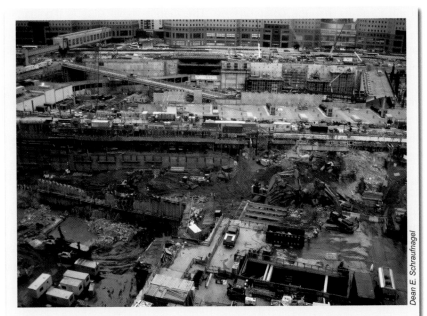

Dean E. Schraufnagel

Large excavations like this one at the World Trade Center site in New York raise and widely disperse soil sediments that contain fungi. Such excavations have the potential to cause large outbreaks of pulmonary fungal infections.

infections in the United States was estimated to be $2.6 billion, approximately 0.24 percent of total U.S. healthcare expenditures (1). That same year, the average added expenditure to treat a patient with a fungal infection in the United States was more than $31,000 above the average annual healthcare expenditure of $4,000 per person (1). Most of this expense was incurred caring for hospitalized patients with invasive aspergillosis, a fungal infection predominantly affecting the lungs (2).

Generally speaking, invasive fungal infections (termed mycoses) can be divided into two broad categories: the opportunistic and the endemic mycoses. Opportunistic fungal infections involve ubiquitous fungi and occur predominantly in individuals whose immune systems are compromised. These infections do not follow any particular geographic distribution and are seen with increasing frequency worldwide. Invasive pulmonary aspergillosis and systemic candidiasis are the most prevalent opportunistic fungal infections. Mold infections that were once considered rare are now emerging as significant infectious complications of the severely immune compromised. The fungus aspergillus is the leading cause of infection-related death in stem cell transplant recipients (3). Allergic lung diseases can also develop in otherwise healthy subjects who are repeatedly exposed to environmental molds.

On the other hand, endemic fungal infections follow distinct geographic distributions that are determined by soil and climate conditions optimal for the fungi's growth. North America is home to three of the major endemic mycoses: histoplasmosis, blastomycosis, and coccidioidomycosis. Their prevalence varies by region.

These three endemic fungal diseases share many characteristics. Illness is acquired by inhaling aerosolized spores. Healthy individuals who contract these diseases generally experience few symptoms, or, if they become ill, recover quickly on their own. In contrast, the infections can be life-threatening in patients with depressed immunity, especially those with acquired immune deficiency syndrome (AIDS) and those receiving immunosuppressive medications. The infections can persist and cause other lung diseases, such as emphysema, to worsen.

What are we learning about lung fungal infections?

Pathophysiology, causes: genetic, environment, microbes

Most pulmonary fungal infections occur after inhalation of fungi that have been aerosolized because their natural habitat was disturbed. Once in the lungs' alveoli (air sacs), the fungus is engulfed by macrophages and other cells involved in the primary immune response. Macrophages are usually able to neutralize and destroy the pathogens that they attack, but many fungi have developed a way to disable the macrophage's weapons, and some fungi have actually developed the ability to grow and multiply inside macrophages.

Secondary or adaptive immunity cells are called to the site of infection, and in healthy individuals, this action can usually control the infection's spread. The fungus is contained, but the sites of initial infection can remain as granulomas, collections of different types of immune cells. The granulomas later degenerate to scars and often calcify. Calcified granulomas may be seen years later on x-ray images.

When cellular immunity is impaired, as it is, for instance, in AIDS, infection with an endemic fungus cannot be controlled. Almost any organ can be involved

Fungal Lung Disease

CASE STUDY

A 66-year-old Indiana woman was hospitalized for an abnormal chest radiograph and respiratory symptoms. Five years earlier, she had been diagnosed with sarcoidosis and treated with an immunosuppressive drug, azathioprine. Three months earlier, infliximab, a new potent anti-cytokine (tumor necrosis factor) immunosuppressive agent, had been started. One month before hospital admission, she developed fever, weakness, shortness of breath, productive cough, nausea, and vomiting, leading to dehydration and a 20-pound weight loss. A chest computed tomography scan showed small nodules scattered in both lungs. She continued to worsen despite many courses of antibacterial antibiotics. In the hospital, her blood pressure dropped. She had fever and a rapid heart rate. Her oxygen level fell and she needed supplemental oxygen. Bronchoscopy with transbronchial biopsy showed granulomas containing the fungus Histoplasma. Urine Histoplasma antigen was positive. She was treated with a potent but potentially toxic antifungal agent, amphotericin B. She improved and was discharged to a long-term care facility after a prolonged hospitalization that was complicated by respiratory failure requiring mechanical ventilation.

Comment

Infection by the fungus Histoplasma capsulatum, or histoplasmosis, is one of the most common infectious complications of medicines that block the inflammatory mediator tumor necrosis factor. Delay in establishing the diagnosis and initiating the appropriate antifungal therapy usually occurs because fungal infections are much less common and harder to diagnose than bacterial pneumonia, which they resemble. Furthermore, the risk of invasive fungal infections in patients receiving anti-cytokine therapy is under-recognized despite the much wider use of these agents today. Delayed diagnosis and treatment can lead to a tragic outcome.

as the infection spreads throughout the body. The presence of structural lung disease, such as emphysema, impairs the clearance of the infection and allows a chronic condition to take hold. White blood cells (especially neutrophils) are critical to fight certain fungal infections such as those due to the fungus *Aspergillus*.

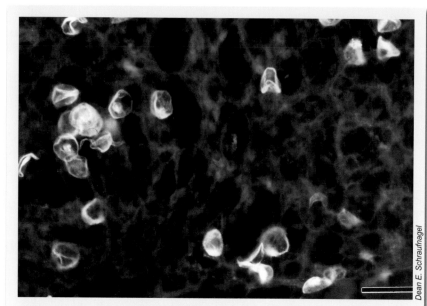

This scanning electron microscopic picture shows the fungus Pneumocystis jiroveci, *which commonly causes pneumonia in persons with AIDS.*

Dean E. Schraufnagel

A number of recent studies suggest that climate changes have disrupted the natural habitat of some endemic fungi, leading to significant changes in their epidemiology. One revealing example is the noticeable increase in the incidence of the fungus coccidioidomycosis, which has been linked to distinct patterns of environmental and climatic change in parts of Arizona between 1998 and 2001. Other examples include the expanding geographic distribution of blastomycosis in the mountains of Northeast Tennessee and the recent outbreak of *Cryptococcus gattii*, a fungus previously associated with tropical and subtropical climates, in the Pacific Northwest.

How are fungal infections prevented, treated, and managed?

Prevention, treatment, staying healthy, prognosis

Despite years of research and much progress in the field, no fungal vaccine is available for clinical use. Today, the most effective way of preventing fungal infections in individuals at risk is by avoiding activities that are associated with exposure to the fungi. Antifungal medication to prevent infection is recommended only in patients with severe immunosuppression, especially since it may lead to the emergence of fungi that are resistant to these medications.

During the last two decades, the number of antifungal agents available for clinical use has increased. Until the mid-1980s, amphotericin B had been the antifungal drug of choice for most fungal infections. At least a half dozen new drugs, which are less toxic than amphotericin B, are now used to treat fungal infections. Amphotericin B is still used in the initial treatment of severe and central nervous system fungal infections. It is usually followed by a maintenance regimen using the new medications.

Immunosuppressed patients should be educated about their risk for developing fungal infections and advised about activities they should avoid, symptoms of fungal disease, and when to report possible exposure or symptoms to their doctor. High-risk activities include demolition and renovation of old buildings, clearing shrubs and debris, and spelunking.

For the most part, treatment of endemic pulmonary fungal infections is very effective, especially when patients are diagnosed and treated in a timely fashion. For the opportunistic fungal infections, the prognosis depends mostly on the immune state of the patient. Therapy is more likely to be effective if immunity is recovered. The most striking example is the impact of anti-retroviral therapy for HIV, which has greatly reduced the incidence and outcome of opportunistic fungal infections in patients infected with HIV.

Are we making a difference?

Research past, present, and future

During the past two decades, research has led to significant advancements in the diagnosis and treatment of fungal infections. Previously, diagnosis was possible only by isolating the organism. Today, urinary and blood tests are used in clinical practice for the rapid diagnosis of invasive fungal infection.

Drug discovery and development have resulted in reformulation of old drugs with a great reduction in toxicity, expansion of individual classes of drugs with better coverage of more fungi, and new classes of drugs with increased efficacy and fewer side effects.

It is now recognized that many fungi that were once routinely dismissed as contaminants are true human pathogens, although mostly for severely immune compromised patients. These include the *zygomycetes* and a variety of molds. Even more worrisome is that several of these organisms are resistant to standard treatment and there is no sensitive diagnostic test. In addition, resistant species of common fungi such as *Candida* and *Aspergillus* are also on the rise.

What we need to cure or eliminate fungal lung disease

Because fungi are everywhere in soil (about 75,000 species have been identified), it is not possible to consider eliminating fungal infections. Although great progress has been made in diagnosing and treating the illnesses they cause, improvement is still needed in all areas. As science gains a better understanding of their basic mechanisms of action, new targets to interrupt the life cycle of the fungi or to strengthen the host immune system are being identified.

The most important immediate step in controlling fungal infections is to increase awareness among clinicians of the significance of these pathogens and the changing patient population at risk. Longer term, it is essential that new diagnostic tests be developed that can provide a rapid and accurate diagnosis, especially for the emerging pathogens. It also will be important to be able to predict their susceptibility to drugs. Researchers must continue to search for novel agents that target key molecular pathways to combat organisms that are resistant to current antifungal therapy. Alterations in the host immune response to fungi could boost clearance of the infection and limit the damage to lung tissue.

Research must also continue to address the interface of the host and fungal pathogen. Knowing how the human host recognizes and counteracts invading fungi and how fungi evade the immune system and survive inside the host cells is important for controlling and eliminating infection. Researchers have identified a number of fungal factors necessary to establish the disease—knowledge of which may eventually lead to a vaccine.

References

1. Wilson LS, Reyes CM, Stolpman M, Speckman J, Allen K, Beney J. The direct cost and incidence of systemic fungal infections. *Value Health* 2002;5:26–34.
2. Dasbach EJ, Davies GM, Teutsch SM. Burden of aspergillosis-related hospitalizations in the United States. *Clin Infect Dis* 2000;31:1524–1528.
3. Ben-Ami R, Lewis RE, Kontoyiannis DP. Invasive mould infections in the setting of hematopoietic cell transplantation: current trends and new challenges. *Curr Opin Infect Dis* 2009;22:376–384.

Web sites of interest

Medline Plus
www.nlm.nih.gov/medlineplus/fungalinfections.html

Centers for Disease Control and Prevention
Division of Bacterial and Mycotic Diseases, Mycotic Diseases Branch
www.cdc.gov/ncidod/dbmd/mdb/goals.htm

Infectious Disease Society of America
www.idsociety.org

possibly because the injurious events continue, or because of defects in the inflammatory or repair processes. When the injurious agent is known, the extent of the injury and time of exposure to the injurious agent are important determinants in disease outcome.

More is known about the interstitial diseases with known causes, such as the occupational exposures. For example, it appears that minerals (for example, asbestos and silica) that cause interstitial lung disease directly injure the lung and cannot be easily eliminated. Thus, ongoing inflammatory and fibrotic reactions occur. In patients with farmer's lung, recurrent exposure to the offending particles (antigens) stimulates the immune system recurrently, which results in fibrosis. A similar recurrent immune stimulation probably occurs with the autoimmune diseases, such as rheumatoid arthritis. For most of the interstitial lung diseases of unknown cause, the mechanisms of lung injury and fibrosis are also unknown. In several interstitial diseases, viral infection has been postulated to be the inciting cause, but this association has not yet been proven.

How is it prevented, treated, and managed?

Prevention, treatment, staying healthy, prognosis

When the cause of the disease is known, the injurious agent should be avoided. For example, with hypersensitivity pneumonitis, one should avoid dust and mold. With idiopathic disorders, because the cause is unknown, there is no known way to prevent them. However, a number of possible risk factors for disease have been reported, and abstaining from cigarette smoking and treating gastroesophageal reflux disease are recommended.

As it has been long thought that inflammation precedes fibrosis, therapeutic regimens for interstitial lung disease have included corticosteroids (for example, prednisone) and immunosuppressive agents (for example, azathioprine and cyclophosphamide). These drugs are helpful in cases of connective tissue–related lung disease and certain other interstitial lung diseases. In patients with severe fibrosis, treatments targeting inflammation, however, have not been shown to improve survival or quality of life. One study did find that patients with IPF treated with high-dose N-acetyl cysteine, an antioxidant, in addition to a standard regimen of corticosteroids and azathioprine had better lung function compared to those on the standard regimen alone (9). Other drugs are being studied.

Lung transplantation is the only option shown to prolong survival in cases of advanced interstitial lung disease, especially IPF, and is possible for patients younger than 65 without other significant medical conditions. However, lung transplantation outcomes remain unsatisfactory, as the five-year survival rate is approximately 40 percent and the median survival is 3.9 years in post-transplant patients with IPF (10). Of those patients with IPF who are waiting to receive a transplant, more than 30 percent die before receiving one. In 2007, IPF surpassed chronic obstructive pulmonary disease as the most common diagnostic group to receive a lung transplant (11), further highlighting the urgent need for effective medical therapies for this and related progressive lung diseases.

Interstitial lung diseases have varying prognoses. Sarcoidosis usually has a good prognosis, with reversal of disease in most cases. On the other hand, IPF, one of the most common interstitial lung diseases, has the worst prognosis, with a median survival of two to three years (2).

Are we making a difference?

Research past, present, and future

An understanding of the mechanisms of the idiopathic forms of interstitial lung disease is only now emerging. Studies of cells in culture and in animals have revealed a number of molecules and molecular pathways (such as transforming growth factor-beta) that promote fibrosis. It appears that an unidentified, probably inhaled, agent may injure the lung and activate cells, such as macrophages and airway lining epithelial cells. The activated cells then produce factors that recruit immune cells into the lung. The immune cells produce or activate sets of molecules that, in turn, activate other molecules to stimulate other cells called fibroblasts to produce and deposit collagen and other connective tissue components, which constitute lung fibrosis.

Studies of the genetic background of patients show that alterations in specific genes (for example, surfactant protein genes and telomerase) may predispose individuals to IPF. Further evidence for the role of genetics in interstitial lung disease comes from studies in patients with other disorders (for example, sarcoidosis and Hermansky–Pudlak syndrome) where mutations in specific genes are associated with a higher incidence of lung fibrosis (12). Further research on these rare diseases caused by a single gene defect may shed light on disease processes that are also important in interstitial lung disease.

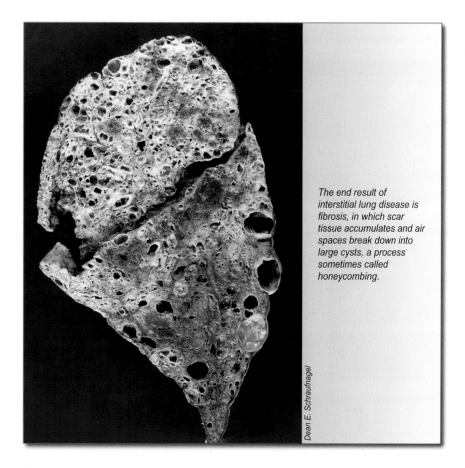

The end result of interstitial lung disease is fibrosis, in which scar tissue accumulates and air spaces break down into large cysts, a process sometimes called honeycombing.

Dean E. Schraufnagel

What do we need to do to cure or eliminate interstitial lung disease?

Although considerable progress has been made in understanding these conditions, curing and eliminating interstitial lung disease is still a distant goal. A clearer understanding of how the cells fail to adequately repair the lung is still needed. Understanding basic mechanisms should lead to better markers to diagnose and follow patients. With these much-needed markers, therapeutic trials will be easier and more cost effective to conduct. Current clinical trials are studying agents that reduce the fibrotic signaling within the lung, reduce pulmonary hypertension associated with interstitial lung disease, and alleviate oxidative stress. These clinical studies are usually coupled with basic science studies to learn more about the mechanisms of disease and to develop biological

ILD has affected many notable Americans

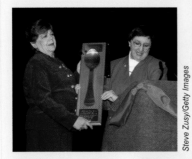
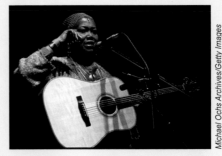
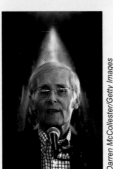
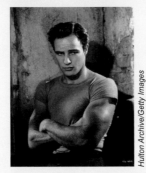
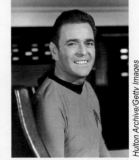

Interstitial lung disease is killing more Americans each year. Former Utah Governor Olene Smith Walker (top left) is living with the disease. Others, unfortunately, have died of the disease, including folk singer and human rights advocate Odetta, writer Peter Benchley (bottom left) and actors Marlon Brando and James Doohan.

markers. To date, trials testing new drugs for the treatment of interstitial lung disease have not been successful or have slowed the progression of disease only modestly, but it is hoped as more is learned about the cells and molecules that are altered in these conditions, the better the chance for success. Both academic centers and pharmaceutical companies are conducting clinical trials to test the safety and effectiveness of several drugs. The National Heart, Lung, and Blood Institute's clinical research network (IPFnet) conducts therapeutic trials in the United States. Recently, stem cells have been considered for therapy, but more needs to be learned before these and other potential therapeutic strategies can be used.

References

1. Coultas DB, Zumwalt RE, Black WC, Sobonya RE. The epidemiology of interstitial lung diseases. *Am J Respir Crit Care Med* 1994;150:967–972.
2. American Thoracic Society. Idiopathic pulmonary fibrosis: diagnosis and treatment. International consensus statement. American Thoracic Society (ATS), and the European Respiratory Society (ERS). *Am J Respir Crit Care Med* 2000;161:646–664.
3. Olson AL, Swigris JJ, Lezotte DC, Norris JM, Wilson CG, Brown KK. Mortality from pulmonary fibrosis increased in the United States from 1992 to 2003. *Am J Respir Crit Care Med* 2007;176:277–284.
4. Mannino DM, Etzel RA, Parrish RG. Pulmonary fibrosis deaths in the United States, 1979–1991. An analysis of multiple-cause mortality data. *Am J Respir Crit Care Med* 1996;153:1548–1552.
5. American Thoracic Society, European Respiratory Society. American Thoracic Society/European Respiratory Society International Multidisciplinary Consensus Classification of the Idiopathic Interstitial Pneumonias. This joint statement of the American Thoracic Society (ATS), and the European Respiratory Society (ERS) was adopted by the ATS board of directors, June 2001 and by the ERS Executive Committee, June 2001. *Am J Respir Crit Care Med* 2002;165:277–304.
6. Raghu G, Weycker D, Edelsberg J, Bradford WZ, Oster G. Incidence and prevalence of idiopathic pulmonary fibrosis. *Am J Respir Crit Care Med* 2006;174:810–816.
7. Gribbin J, Hubbard RB, Le Jeune I, Smith CJ, West J, Tata LJ. Incidence and morality of idiopathic pulmonary fibrosis and sarcoidosis in the UK. *Thorax* 2006;61:980–985.
8. Armanios MY, Chen JJ, Cogan JD, Alder JK, Ingersoll RG, Markin C, Lawson WE, Xie M, Vulto I, Phillips JA 3rd, et al. Telomerase mutations in families with idiopathic pulmonary fibrosis. *N Engl J Med* 2007;356:1317–1326.
9. Demedts M, Behr J, Buhl R, Costabel U, Dekhuijzen R, Jansen HM, MacNee W, Thomeer M, Wallaert B, Laurent F, et al. High-dose acetylcysteine in idiopathic pulmonary fibrosis. *N Engl J Med* 2005;353:2229–2242.
10. Trulock EP, Christie JD, Edwards LB, Boucek MM, Aurora P, Taylor DO, Dobbels F, Rahmel AO, Keck BM, Hertz MI. Registry of the International Society for Heart and Lung Transplantation: twenty-fourth official adult lung and heart-lung transplantation report–2007. *J Heart Lung Transplant* 2007;26:782–795.
11. McCurry KR, Shearon TH, Edwards LB, et al. Lung transplantation in the United States, 1998–2007. *Am J Transplant* 2009;9:942–958.
12. Steele MP, Brown KK. Genetic predisposition to respiratory diseases: infiltrative lung diseases. *Respiration* 2007;74:601–608.

Web sites of interest

ATS/ERS Consensus Statement on Idiopathic Pulmonary Fibrosis
http://thoracic.org/statements

NIH Clinical trials
www.clinicaltrials.gov

Coalition of Pulmonary Fibrosis
www.coalitionforpf.org

Children's Interstitial Lung Disease Foundation, Inc.
www.childfoundation.us/

Pulmonary Fibrosis Foundation
www.pulmonaryfibrosis.org

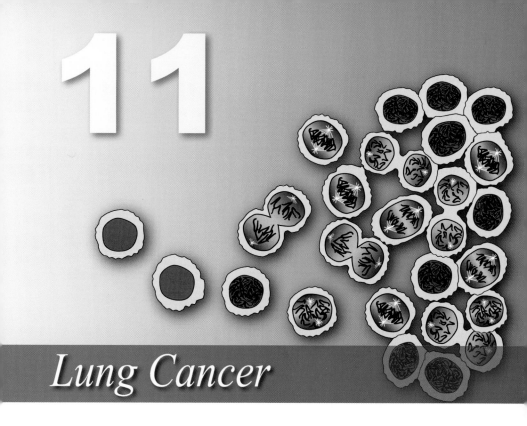

Lung Cancer

Lung cancer is the deadliest of all cancers in the United States and the world. It kills more Americans than the next four most common cancers combined. Lung cancer is largely preventable; inroads in reducing cigarette smoking are having a positive influence, though other environmental exposures also put people at risk. Advances in understanding this disease are leading to new means of diagnosis and treatment.

Whom does it affect?

Epidemiology, prevalence, economic burden, vulnerable populations

The World Health Organization's Global Burden of Disease analysis projects 1,676,000 deaths from lung cancer worldwide in 2015. It predicts that this toll will continue to rise to reach a staggering 2,279,000 deaths in the year 2030 (1). In the United States, it has been estimated that 159,390 individuals (70,490 women and 88,900 men) died from lung cancer in 2009—more deaths than from cancers of the breast, colon, pancreas, and prostate combined (2).

Lung cancer is a disease of modern times. At the turn of the 20th century, lung cancer was rare, accounting for less than 0.5 percent of all malignancies.

Lung and bronchus deaths by state, 2009

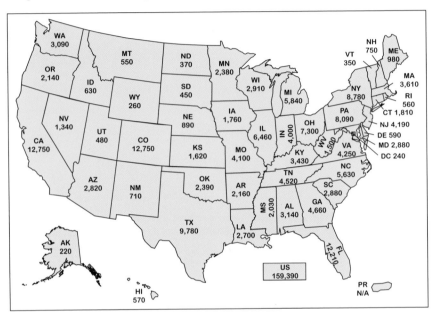

Lung cancer is the leading cause of cancer death in the United States. Its low survival rates are due in part to the lack of a method to detect it early. American Cancer Society. *Cancer Facts and Figures 2009.* Atlanta: American Cancer Society; 2009.

In the early decades of the 1900s, a steeply rising incidence of lung cancer in men led to speculation implicating a variety of etiologies, including tuberculosis, influenza, industrial pollution, and chronic bronchitis, among others. In that period, tobacco tar liberated from burning tobacco was found to be carcinogenic, and clinical observations suggested a link between cigarette smoking and lung cancer. In 1950, landmark epidemiologic studies published in the United States and in the United Kingdom demonstrated that an association between cigarette smoking and lung cancer existed, that intensity of smoking was a factor in the development of lung cancer, and that a lag time of years between exposure to cigarette smoking and diagnosis of lung cancer was typical. In 1964, the United States Surgeon General issued a landmark report on the health consequences of smoking that acknowledged the causative role of cigarette smoking in the development of lung cancer.

CASE STUDY

A 65-year-old man had a dry cough for several months. He had smoked one pack of cigarettes a day for 35 years and quit five years earlier. He had a history of chronic obstructive pulmonary disease (COPD). A chest radiograph showed a mass in the left lower lobe with lymph node enlargement. A chest computed tomography (CT) scan confirmed these findings. A positron emission tomography (PET) scan showed abnormalities in the mass and lymph nodes, but no other areas. Magnetic resonance imaging (MRI) of the brain was normal. A bronchoscopy with endobronchial ultrasound confirmed lung cancer, with adenocarcinoma histology. The cancer was staged by its size and spread as T2aN2M0, clinical stage IIIA. (T is for tumor size and location; N is for lymph node spread; and M is for distant metastasis.)

Comment

Lung cancer symptoms typically include persistent cough, difficulty breathing, coughing up blood, and chest discomfort, though many patients are asymptomatic. Patients with advanced disease often have weight loss, fatigue, or pain outside the chest. This patient's evaluation included diagnostic studies generally performed in a lung cancer evaluation, the purpose of which is to determine the cancer stage. Staging predicts prognosis and influences treatment.

Before 1950, lung cancer in women was still an uncommon occurrence. However, over the latter half of the 20th century, an epidemic of lung cancer in women occurred, mirroring the rapid rise of lung cancer among men witnessed earlier. Since 1988, lung cancer has killed more women than breast cancer each year in the United States. Since 1991, lung cancer mortality rates have been declining in men, while in women they appear to be plateauing. Lung cancer is unfortunately likely to remain the leading cause of cancer death in both men and women in this country for the near future.

The economic burden of lung cancer to the nation is immense, and can be gauged in a number of ways, including estimation of life-years lost, costs associated with premature deaths, and direct costs of medical care. In 2005 in the

United States, lung cancer caused 2.4 million person-years-of-life-lost (person-years-of-life-lost is the difference between the actual age at death due to disease and the expected age of death). For this statistic, lung cancer far exceeds any other type of cancer (3). The economic costs associated with those lost years of life are substantial. One study estimated that those costs in 2000 in the United States were $289.4 billion (4). Direct medical costs related to treatment for lung cancer are also staggering. In 2004, the National Cancer Institute estimated lung cancer treatment expenditures at $9.6 billion (3).

Unfortunately, because of the lack of effective screening technology, only about a third of patients are identified at an early stage. Most patients do not seek medical attention until the disease is advanced, and at that point, treatment is of limited success. Overall survival is poor.

What we are learning about the disease

Epidemiology, prevalence, economic burden, vulnerable populations

The pathophysiology of lung cancer is best described as a "multi-hit" event. Carcinogens, most commonly those in cigarette smoke but also including many different environmental exposures, can result in DNA damage or mutation. The cumulative effect of several "hits" may result in irreversible effects on the biologic mechanisms that control growth, proliferation, vascular supply, and death of normal cells. Collective dysregulation of these mechanisms is felt to lead to lung cancer.

Many factors affect lung cancer risk, but cigarette smoking has been the largest single factor contributing to the dramatic rise in lung cancer rates in the United States. Since the 1964 Surgeon General's report on the health consequences of smoking, the yearly per capita consumption of cigarettes in the United States has declined. Nonetheless, almost one quarter of Americans continue to smoke, which makes it likely that lung cancer will remain the most important cancer in this country for years to come. Cigar and pipe smoking also increase risk, but less so than cigarettes.

While it is certainly one of the greatest risk factors for lung cancer, tobacco smoking is not the *only* risk factor. An estimated 15 percent of lung cancers in women in the United States and a much larger percentage of lung cancers in women in Asia occur in non-smokers. Epidemiologic studies show that in the

United States, smoking is responsible for 90 percent of lung cancer cases, occupational exposures to carcinogens cause 9 to 15 percent of cases, and radon accounts for 10 percent of cases (5). (The sum of these risk estimates exceeds 100 percent because many individuals have multiple risk factors, and these factors are synergistic.)

A number of occupational carcinogens have been defined, including asbestos, benzopyrene, arsenic, chromium, and nickel. High doses of radiation increase lung cancer risk. Radon and its decay products are associated with lung cancer in miners exposed to high levels of radon gas and are of concern because of the potential exposure in domestic environments. Other factors known to influence lung cancer risk include air pollution, the presence of other lung diseases, such as COPD and interstitial lung disease, and exposure to environmental tobacco smoke. Diet has also been implicated. Case-control and prospective studies have generally found that diets rich in fruits and vegetables are associated with lower risk for lung cancer.

Finally, genetic susceptibility also plays a role in lung cancer. Many studies have shown that a history of lung cancer in a first-degree relative is associated with increased risk, and that this association may be of more significance in younger individuals. Genetically determined host factors may be important at many points in the cumulative steps leading to lung cancer, including the risk of nicotine dependence, carcinogen metabolic detoxification, activation of carcinogens, and the processes of DNA damage and repair.

How is it prevented, treated, and managed?

Prevention, treatment, staying healthy, prognosis

Most lung cancer risk factors are modifiable and, therefore, can be minimized or eliminated. Cigarette smoking, occupational exposures, radon exposure, and environmental tobacco smoke all can be reduced. Cigarette smoking cessation at any age will decrease lung cancer risk. Though it never reaches the level of a never-smoker, the risk of lung cancer in an individual who quits smoking decreases with longer duration of abstinence. Community and public health initiatives increasingly limit exposure to second-hand smoke. Government regulation has reduced occupational exposure to most carcinogens.

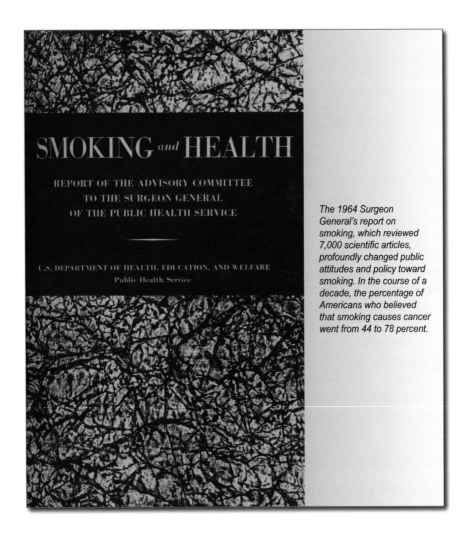

SMOKING *and* HEALTH

REPORT OF THE ADVISORY COMMITTEE
TO THE SURGEON GENERAL
OF THE PUBLIC HEALTH SERVICE

U.S. DEPARTMENT OF HEALTH, EDUCATION, AND WELFARE
Public Health Service

The 1964 Surgeon General's report on smoking, which reviewed 7,000 scientific articles, profoundly changed public attitudes and policy toward smoking. In the course of a decade, the percentage of Americans who believed that smoking causes cancer went from 44 to 78 percent.

Treatment for lung cancer is typically guided by stage, although individual factors, such as overall health and coexisting medical conditions, are important. Complete surgical removal is the best treatment, but it is only possible in patients with early stage disease. Chemotherapy is beneficial at most stages of disease, although it and radiation therapy are curative in only a minority of patients. Palliative therapy can improve the quality and often the length of life. A multidisciplinary approach that incorporates medical, surgical, and social support services generally renders the best care.

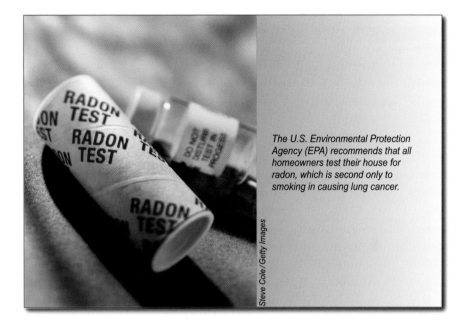

The U.S. Environmental Protection Agency (EPA) recommends that all homeowners test their house for radon, which is second only to smoking in causing lung cancer.

Steve Cole/Getty Images

Are we making a difference?

Research past, present, and future

Epidemiologic research has vastly improved our understanding of lung cancer risk factors and found them to be modifiable with appropriate interventions. Lung cancer is much less common in persons without identifiable risk factors. Applying this information to develop and implement prevention strategies has led to decreased smoking, which is now associated with a declining lung cancer rate in men and a plateauing rate in women in the United States. These data have induced legislative efforts to regulate tobacco and eliminate exposure to cigarette smoke in public areas. Although these regulations have already decreased the incidence of heart disease, it will take years to assess their impact on lung cancer.

Lung cancer research seeks to improve methods for early diagnosis; understand genetic and molecular factors that influence carcinogenesis, tumor behavior, and outcomes; develop new treatments based on sound scientific knowledge; and individualize treatment based on patient situations and a better understanding of tumor biology.

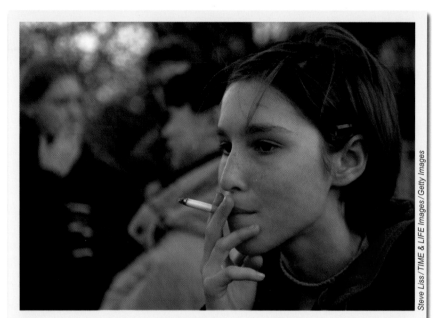

Although smoking has decreased among all teenagers, girls are now slightly more likely to smoke than boys.

There is unfortunately no reliable screening tool for early lung cancer detection. Screening studies have failed to show a clear increase in survival in high-risk patients. The National Lung Screening Trial is an ongoing, large, prospective study comparing yearly screening chest radiographs versus yearly screening computed tomography scans in persons at risk for lung cancer because of smoking. This study should increase our understanding of whether either of these means of early detection will decrease lung cancer mortality.

The ability to study the entire genome now makes it possible to understand genetic variation not only between those with and without the disease, but also among those with different severities of illness. These studies also may give insight into the mechanism of disease and lead to potential therapeutic targets. For example, several studies have reported an association between lung cancer and a single genetic variant on chromosome 15. This site includes genes that code nicotinic acetylcholine receptors that are strongly associated with smoking behavior. Although the genetic risk alone for lung cancer is relatively small (it increases incidence by two- to three-fold), it may be magnified by interaction with environmental influences.

Finding changes in the molecular pathways that regulate cell proliferation, programmed cell death (apoptosis), new blood vessel development (angiogenesis), invasion, and metastasis are critical to developing new treatments. A breakthrough in this area came with the discovery of the epidermal growth factor receptor (EGFR) signaling pathway, which is involved in many processes of human lung cancers.

Molecular characterization of EGFR has facilitated description of its mutations, as well as the ability to identify the number of copies of the EGFR gene and quantification of its protein expression in malignant tissue. This has enabled patients' tissues to be tested and classified with regard to EGFR mutational status. Specific inhibitors of the EGFR pathway have been developed for treatment of lung cancer. Selected EGFR mutations, high EGFR gene copy number, and EGFR protein over-expression have been reported to be predictive of response to treatment with EGFR antagonists.

Therapeutic agents targeted to the EGFR pathway have been developed by the following strategies: 1) block the binding of the factor to the outside of the cell, 2) inactivate the receptor with anti-EGFR antibodies, and 3) block the intracellular effects of the signaling pathway with small molecules before they trigger action in the cell.

The genetic profile associated with response to medical therapy against EGFR includes Asian heritage, female sex, nonsmoking status, and adenocarcinoma cell type, although benefit also may be observed in individuals without these characteristics. The ability to target therapy based on molecular characteristics of an individual tumor represents an enormous advance in treatment and an important step toward the goal of personalized lung cancer care.

What we need to cure or eliminate lung cancer

Steps to reduce and eliminate lung cancer began with the understanding of the central role of tobacco in this disease. Public awareness campaigns that reduce smoking and strong legislative action to eliminate tobacco smoke in public places and further decrease in cigarette use are saving lives. Attention to other risk factors, such as radon, should also diminish lung cancer incidence.

Early diagnosis is an important factor in survival and would be greatly facilitated by identifying a simple marker of lung cancer. Because the lung is a difficult organ to sample, a blood test, swabs for cells in the mouth, or exhaled breath are being explored as surrogate indicators. It is hoped that reliably identifying cells and molecules that predict cancer could allow screening that would lead to early diagnoses and saved lives. Refinements of viewing and sampling cells of the bronchi and lung are providing improved and less invasive diagnostic techniques. New bronchoscopic technologies using ultrasound and electromagnetic navigation may improve the chance of making a correct diagnosis when the cancer is confined to a small area of the lung. The importance of this is underscored because a small lung cancer diagnosed early is more likely to be able to be completely surgically removed and has a better chance of cure.

Identifying genetic predisposition to lung cancer could increase the accuracy and efficacy of screening. Genetic predisposition to lung cancer may be related to variations within genes that are associated with controlling the growth cycle of the cell, its metabolism of carcinogens, and DNA repair. The search for markers explores genes differentially expressed in patients with lung cancer compared to those without. Gene expression profiling on bronchial cells suggests that such biomarkers may predict lung cancer risk.

In the future, molecular approaches will likely allow selection of patients who are most likely to benefit from specific therapies, and will guide the development of more effective therapeutic agents. The potential for research in this area is enormous, as these approaches should also improve the ability to predict individual patient outcomes.

Lung cancer staging is defined by clinical outcomes and, at present, is based solely on anatomic factors—the size of the tumor and where it has spread. Accurate staging is the basis for predicting survival and is key to clinical trials that compare treatments among homogeneous populations of patients. For example, patients with Stage I non-small cell lung cancer treated with surgical resection have a five-year survival of about 73 percent (6). Considering these are early stage patients, this five-year survival is lower than expected; clearly some patients do poorly despite surgery. If those patients could be identified, further treatment would be given to try to improve their survival. Current genetic research has identified several genes that may predict outcomes for patients. Genes linked to lung cancer, and in particular to poor survival, are being systematically cataloged. Further study should clarify which genes and gene products will predict patient outcomes. This may help identify individuals who would benefit from more aggressive treatment, and which genes might be targets for new therapies.

All of these investigative efforts will enhance our understanding of the molecular mechanisms governing carcinogenesis and tumor behavior. Translation of this knowledge to the development of biomarkers predicting risk, clinical models that can more accurately predict patient outcomes, and novel therapies targeted to molecular pathways of carcinogenesis will facilitate the goal of personalized treatment for individual patients with lung cancer.

References

1. World Health Organization Web site. Projections of mortality and burden of disease, 2002–2030. Available at: http://www.who.int/healthinfo/global_burden_disease/projections2002/en/. Accessed January 30, 2010.
2. Jemal A, Siegel R, Ward E, Hao Y, Xu J, Thun MJ. Cancer statistics, 2009. *CA Cancer J Clin* 2009;59:225–249.
3. National Cancer Institute Web site. Cancer trends progress report - 2007 update. Available at: http://progressreport.cancer.gov. Accessed January 30, 2010.
4. Yabroff KR, Bradley CJ, Mariotto AB, Brown ML, Feuer EJ. Estimates and projections of value of life lost from cancer deaths in the United States. *J Natl Cancer Inst* 2008;100: 1755–1762.
5. Alberg AJ, Ford JG, Samet JM. 2007. Epidemiology of lung cancer: ACCP evidence-based clinical practice guidelines (2nd edition). *Chest* 132(3 Suppl):29S-55S.
6. Goldstraw P, Crowley J, Chansky K, Giroux DJ, Groome PA, Rami-Porta R, Postmus PE, Rusch V, Sobin L. 2007. The IASLC Lung Cancer Staging Project: proposals for the revision of the TNM stage groupings in the forthcoming (seventh) edition of the TNM Classification of malignant tumours. *J Thorac Oncol* 2(8):706–714.

Web sites of interest

National Cancer Institute
Lung Cancer
www.cancer.gov/cancertopics/types/lung

Medline Plus
Lung Cancer
www.nlm.nih.gov/medlineplus/lungcancer.html

American Cancer Society
www.cancer.org

National Lung Cancer Partnership
www.nationallungcancerpartnership.org/

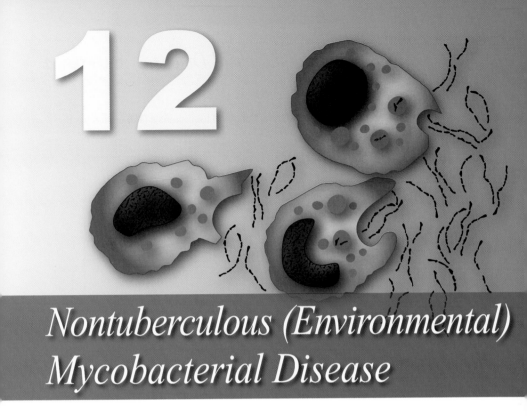

Nontuberculous (Environmental) Mycobacterial Disease

Nontuberculous mycobacteria (NTM) are in the same family as the organisms that cause tuberculosis and leprosy, but unlike those organisms, NTM are widely dispersed in our environment, vary greatly in their ability to cause disease, and are not spread from person to person. There are about 140 different species of mycobacteria. Mycobacteria not closely related to tuberculosis or leprosy are called *nontuberculous mycobacteria*, *environmental mycobacteria*, and *mycobacteria other than tuberculosis* (MOTT). Recent studies have documented increases in NTM infections, and, in many areas of the United States, these infections outnumber tuberculosis.

Whom does it affect?

Epidemiology, prevalence, economic burden, vulnerable populations

Nontuberculous mycobacteria were first identified in the late 19th century, when a tuberculosis-like disease was reported in chickens. In the 1930s, they were documented to cause disease in humans, but it was not until the 1950s that pulmonary disease due to these organisms became more commonly recognized. Most clinicians discounted the clinical significance of these bacteria, until the acquired

Nontuberculous mycobacterial (NTM) infections and tuberculosis (TB) case rates in Ontario, 1997–2003

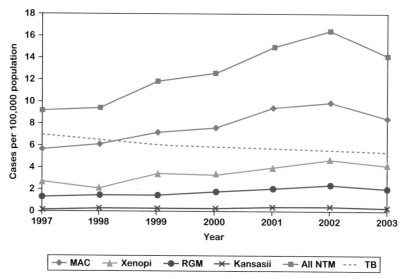

Nontuberculous mycobacterial disease has increased significantly in recent years (all P < .001). These Canadian data most likely mirror U.S. data. The rates are calculated from the total number of cases and population data from Statistics Canada (available at: http://www.statcan.ca/english/Pgdb/demo02.htm). MAC, Mycobacterium avium complex; RGM, rapidly growing mycobacteria; kansasii and xenopi are species of mycobacteria. Reproduced from Isolation prevalence of pulmonary non-tuberculous mycobacteria in Ontario, 1997–2003, Thorax, Marras TK, Chedore P, Ying AM, Jamieson F 62 661–666, 2007 with permission from BMJ Publishing Group Ltd.

immune deficiency syndrome (AIDS) epidemic, when patients with advanced human immunodeficiency virus (HIV) disease began developing mycobacterial infections that spread throughout their bodies. The subsequent development of new antimicrobials demonstrated that these infections could be treated and prevented in individuals with HIV. Fortunately, the discovery of potent antiretroviral drugs has improved the immune systems of patients with AIDS and reduced the incidence of mycobacterial infections in these persons. However, pulmonary NTM infections in people uninfected with HIV appear to be increasing.

Determining the number of environmental mycobacterial infections in the United States is difficult because reporting these infections to public health departments is not required. Survey data from state laboratories in the early 1980s estimated the prevalence of NTM infections to be 1 to 2 cases per 100,000 population (1). A similar survey from 1993–1996 reported an annual case rate of

7 to 8 per 100,000. A recent population-based study from Ontario, Canada, documented an increase in the frequency of environmental mycobacterial infections from 9.1 per 100,000 in 1997 to 14.1 per 100,000 in 2003, an annual increase of 8.4 percent (2). Because these infections require therapy that generally lasts two to three times longer than that used to treat tuberculosis, and because recurrences are more common, the prevalence of nontuberculous mycobacterial infections in Ontario has been estimated to be 14 to 35 per 100,000, three to eight times that of tuberculosis (3).

Nontuberculous mycobacterial infections also appear to be increasing in the United States. Studies measuring skin test reactivity found that exposure to the most common environmental mycobacteria, *Mycobacterium avium,* occurs in over 50 percent of adults in the southeastern United States, compared to about 20 percent in other regions of the country (4). The frequency of positive skin test reactions increased from the 1970s to the 1990s, suggesting increased exposure over that period (5). In recent skin test studies, factors that predicted a positive reaction included being male, African American, and born outside the United States, as well as degree of exposure to soil (5,6). However, these factors do not necessarily indicate who will develop mycobacterial disease.

There is one published report describing the economic burden of NTM infections (6a). This report noted that the treatment costs were comparable to other chronic infectious diseases such as HIV/AIDS. Whereas tuberculosis is treated with multiple drugs for six months, most NTM lung infections require 18 to 24 months of treatment. The cost of treatment per patient is probably three or four times that of treating tuberculosis.

While anyone can develop a mycobacterial infection, most patients have underlying structural lung disease, such as chronic obstructive pulmonary disease, cystic fibrosis, bronchiectasis, prior tuberculosis, or chronic aspiration (1). Earlier studies noted a male preponderance in patients with pulmonary disease, but more recent reports have found a female preponderance (7,8). Among women with pulmonary infections, there is often a constellation of physical findings: bronchiectasis, thin body habitus, curvature of the spine (scoliosis), hollowed chest (pectus excavatum), lax heart valve struts (mitral valve prolapse), and joint hypermobility (8,9). The reason for these associations has not been determined and, to date, no significant immunological abnormality has been identified.

CASE STUDY

A 67-year-old woman saw her primary care physician for a chronic cough that was accompanied by fatigue and weight loss. In the previous five years, she had been treated for multiple episodes of "bronchitis" and improved with each treatment, only to have her cough return. The patient had been healthy most of her life with no significant medical problems, and she never smoked. A chest radiograph showed mild lung changes near her heart. A chest computed tomography (CT) scan demonstrated that these abnormalities were due to bronchiectasis and that she had many small nodules consistent with an infection. Although she was unable to produce sputum on her own, specimens were obtained by having her inhale saline, and these specimens eventually grew M. avium complex (MAC) in two of three cultures after about three weeks. Because of her chronic symptoms, abnormal radiograph, and multiple positive cultures, she was begun on a three-drug treatment regimen with plans to treat for approximately 18 months. She improved with the treatment, and by the end of therapy, the organism could no longer be detected in her sputum.

Comment

The lung is the most common site of NTM infections, but lymph nodes, skin, and soft tissue in several areas of the body can also be involved. Patients with pulmonary infections usually have chronic cough, fatigue, malaise, and weight loss. In many instances, patients are misdiagnosed as having chronic bronchitis and treated repeatedly with short courses of antibiotics. Simply isolating the organisms from a respiratory specimen does not mean that the patient has mycobacterial disease.

For years, the term colonization *was used to differentiate those who had no evidence of progressive disease from those who did. For persons considered to be "colonized" with environmental mycobacteria, no treatment was prescribed. However, it is now apparent that many of the patients who were thought to have been "colonized," did, in fact, have evidence of disease on CT scans and had slow progression. To help clinicians with the difficult task of trying to determine if an NTM species is or is not causing disease, the American Thoracic Society and Infectious Diseases Society of America developed a set of criteria that use clinical, radiographic, and microbiologic parameters to distinguish disease from colonization (1).*

What are we learning about this disease?

Pathophysiology, causes: genetic, environment, microbes

The source of NTM infections appears to be environmental exposure, with no person-to-person transmission reported. These mycobacteria are dispersed widely in nature and have been isolated from natural and treated water as well as soil.

Although exposure is common, disease is unusual. The importance of host immunity in resisting infections has been demonstrated in persons with HIV, persons taking immunosuppressive drugs, and those who have mutations of genes that produce proteins of the immune system. These patients usually develop severe mycobacterial infections, including disseminated disease. No genetic predisposition to pulmonary disease, however, has been discovered.

A unique clinical presentation is that of hypersensitivity pneumonitis or "hot-tub lung." In this condition, exposure to environmental mycobacteria in contaminated water can result in an inflammatory response in the lung that can be quite serious. These patients experience shortness of breath and have diffuse abnormalities on their chest radiographs.

NTM are traditionally divided into slowly and rapidly growing organisms, although all grow much slower than most other bacteria. They display a wide range of ability to cause disease (pathogenicity): some species do not cause

Some common slowly and rapidly growing nontuberculous mycobacteria causing pulmonary infections

Slowly growing mycobacteria	Rapidly growing mycobacteria
M. avium	M. abscessus
M. intracellulare	M. chelonae
M. kansasii	M. fortuitum
M. malmoense	
M. simiae	
M. szulgai	
M. xenopi	

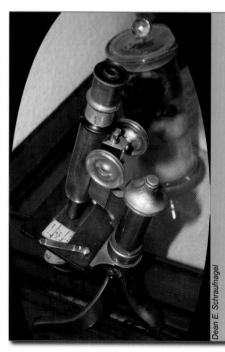

Through this microscope, Robert Koch was the first to view the mycobacteria that cause tuberculosis. He also found mycobacteria in animals and other environments and noted differences in their appearances that brought forth the concept that not all mycobacteria cause tuberculosis.

Dean E. Schraufnagel

disease in humans, some produce disease occasionally, and others almost always cause disease if they are found in sputum. The reason for this variation in pathogenicity is not known. Keeping track of the many different mycobacterial species and which ones are likely to cause disease can be daunting for clinicians.

How is it prevented, treated, and managed?

Prevention, treatment, staying healthy, prognosis

An effective strategy for preventing pulmonary NTM infections is lacking. Except in the case of "hot-tub lung," where ceasing exposure to contaminated water can result in resolution of the condition, it is unknown how to prevent these infections. NTM have been isolated from public water supplies and pose a sterilization problem because they tolerate high water temperature and are resistant to standard decontamination methods.

Although antituberculous drugs have been used widely to prevent the development of tuberculosis, such therapy for NTM is only recommended in patients with advanced HIV disease. Unfortunately, there is no vaccine available for the prevention of environmental mycobacterial infections. There are, however, several reports that the vaccine for tuberculosis, Bacille Calmette-Guerin (BCG), offers some protection against NTM infection in children.

The treatment of environmental mycobacterial infections is almost always more complicated than the treatment of tuberculosis. The drugs, frequency of administration, and duration of therapy will vary depending on the species of NTM causing the disease, site of infection, and extent of disease. Although some antituberculous drugs are also active against NTM, treatment of most infections also requires antibiotics that are not typically used to treat tuberculosis. The treatment may depend on laboratory tests of antibiotic resistance of the isolate causing disease. Prolonged courses of intravenous or inhaled antibiotic therapy may be required.

The prognosis for pulmonary infections due to environmental mycobacteria is variable and depends on many factors, including the specific species involved and its drug susceptibility pattern, extent of disease, presence of other medical problems, and whether or not the patient can tolerate the treatment regimen. For example, the cure rate for disease caused by *M. kansasii* is virtually 100 percent, while that for diseases caused by *M. avium* is 30 to 85 percent. A cure is seldom achieved in patients with pulmonary *M. abscessus* infection (1).

Are we making a difference?

Research past, present, and future

Compared to other lung diseases, relatively little progress has been made in understanding, preventing, or treating disease due to NTM. Although these organisms can be isolated from the environment, it is not clear when and where exposures occur and why some people develop infection but most do not. Few clinical trials have been performed, and most have been small, non-randomized, and uncontrolled. Based on these trials, however, recurrence rates with pulmonary disease appear to be high. Whether this high recurrence is due to failure of the recommended treatment regimens or re-infection with another strain is not clear.

Information is emerging from basic science research. The nature of the different mycobacterial species, their requirements for growth, and their adaptation to different environments are being learned. Individuals with defects in their immune systems are more susceptible to NTM, and the nature of this susceptibility gives

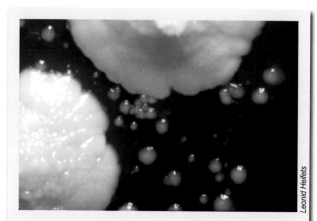

Leonid Heifets

The different species of mycobacteria can be identified based on several factors, such as their appearance when grown in laboratory media. The larger, rough-looking colonies are Mycobacterium chelonae, and the smaller, smooth colonies are Mycobacterium avium.

insights into the immune responses that control the disease. The ability of mycobacteria to live in biofilm may partly explain how they survive in the mucus of the airways of patients with bronchiectasis in the presence of antibiotics.

What we need to cure or eliminate nontuberculous mycobacterial infections

The recently documented increase in NTM infections should be a stimulus to develop better diagnostic tests and discover new drug therapies. Large-scale randomized clinical trials are needed to discover which drugs are best, how long patients should be treated, and which combinations will decrease drug-related toxicity. A better understanding of the transmission and pathogenesis of these increasingly common infections may allow prevention of harm from these ubiquitous environmental bacteria.

Only some of the extensive research on *M. tuberculosis* can be applied to the environmental mycobacteria, but breakthroughs in tuberculosis may be adaptable to other mycobacterial diseases. For example, a blood test similar to the one used for the diagnosis of tuberculosis could be developed. Medications and vaccines being developed for tuberculosis could be tested in NTM disease. There is an urgent need, however, to develop tools for these diseases on their own.

References

1. Griffith DE, Aksamit T, Brown-Elliot BA, Catanzaro A, Daley C, Gordin F, Holland SM, Horsburgh R, Huitt G, Iademarco MF, et al, for the ATS Mycobacterial Diseases Subcommittee; American Thoracic Society; Infectious Disease Society of America. An official ATS/IDSA statement: diagnosis, treatment, and prevention of nontuberculous mycobacterial diseases. *Am J Respir Crit Care Med* 2007;175:367–416.
2. Marras TK, Chedore P, Ying AM, Jamieson F. Isolation prevalence of pulmonary nontuberculous mycobacteria in Ontario, 1997–2003. *Thorax* 2007;62:661–666.
3. Iseman MD, Marras TK. The importance of nontuberculous mycobacterial lung disease. *Am J Respir Crit Care Med* 2008;178:999–1000.
4. Edwards FG. Disease caused by 'atypical' (opportunist) mycobacteria: a whole population review. *Tubercle* 1970;51:285–295.
5. Khan K, Wang J, Marras TK. Nontuberculous mycobacterial sensitization in the United States: national trends over three decades. *Am J Respir Crit Care Med* 2007;176:306–313.
6. Reed C, von Reyn F, Chamblee S, Ellerbrock TV, Johnson JW, Marsh BJ, Johnson LS, Trenschel RJ, Horsburgh CR Jr. Environmental risk factors for infection with *Mycobacterium avium* complex. *Am J Epidemiol* 2006;164:32–40. 6a. Ballarino GJ, Olivier KN, Claypool RJ, Holland SM, Prevots DR. Pulmonary nontuberculous mycobacterial infections: antibiotic treatment and associated costs. Respir Med 2009;103:1448–1455.
7. Iseman MD, Buschman DL, Ackerson LM. Pectus excavatum and scoliosis. Thoracic anomalies associated with pulmonary disease caused by *Mycobacterium avium* complex. *Am Rev Respir Dis* 1991;144:914–916.
8. Prince DS, Peterson DD, Steiner RM, Gottlieb JE, Scott R, Israel HL, Figueroa WG, Fish JE. Infection with *Mycobacterium avium* complex in patients without predisposing conditions. *N Engl J Med* 1989;321:863–868.
9. Kim RD, Greenberg DE, Ehrmantraut ME, Guide SV, Ding L, Shea Y, Brown MR, Chernick M, Steagall WK, Glasgow CG, et al. Pulmonary nontuberculous mycobacterial disease: prospective study of a distinct preexisting syndrome. *Am J Respir Crit Care Med* 2008;178:1066–1074.

Web sites of interest

American Thoracic Society
An Official ATS/IDSA Statement: Diagnosis, Treatment, and Prevention of Nontuberculous Mycobacterial Diseases
www.thoracic.org/statements/resources/mtpi/nontuberculous-mycobacterial-diseases.pdf

National Jewish Health
www.nationaljewish.org

NTM Info & Research, Inc.
www.ntminfo.com

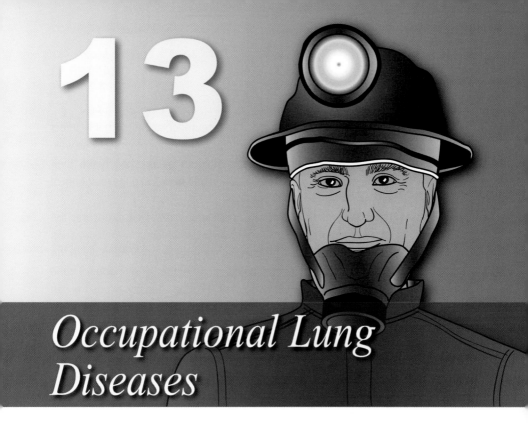

13

Occupational Lung Diseases

Occupational lung diseases are a broad group of diagnoses caused by the inhalation of dusts, chemicals, or proteins. "Pneumoconiosis" is the term used for the diseases associated with inhaling mineral dusts. The severity of the disease is related to the material inhaled and the intensity and duration of the exposure. Even individuals who do not work in the industry can develop occupational disease through indirect exposure. Although these diseases have been documented as far back as ancient Greece and Rome, the incidence of the disease increased dramatically with the development of modern industry.

Whom does it affect?

Epidemiology, prevalence, economic burden, vulnerable populations

In most cases, these diseases are man-made, resulting from inorganic dust exposure during mining, processing, or manufacturing. In New York and New Jersey in the 1970s, asbestosis could be diagnosed in over 70 percent of asbestos insulation workers with greater than 20 years of exposure (1). After the introduction of regulatory agencies and promulgation of dust regulations and their enforcement, these high prevalence rates and others dropped dramatically. For instance, the prevalence of coal workers' pneumoconiosis dropped to 5 percent among miners with greater than 25 years' exposure (1). The pneumoconioses primarily affect those exposed at work, but environmental exposure can make others sick as well. Asbestos insulators expose their wives and children by bringing home their asbestos-covered clothing, and asbestos factories and mines expose residents of nearby neighborhoods.

Different exposures result in different diseases. With silica exposure, the classic and most common disease is chronic silicosis, which develops decades after exposure and is characterized by the silicotic nodule, predominantly in the upper lobes of the lungs, and "eggshell" calcification of the lymph nodes. These findings do not always have clinical symptoms. Higher intensity exposure can result in accelerated or acute silicosis, in which symptoms develop much earlier. Acute silicosis is the least frequent, but it also has the highest mortality rate. The accelerated and chronic forms of silicosis can become complicated silicosis or progressive massive fibrosis, in which the silicotic nodules coalesce into larger lesions in the upper lobes of the lung, and the patients develop increasing breathing difficulty.

Silicosis increases susceptibility to tuberculosis anywhere from 2- to 30-fold. There also is an association between silicosis and immune-mediated diseases, such as systemic sclerosis and rheumatoid arthritis, which may develop with silica exposure alone. Systemic lupus erythematosus has been linked to acute and accelerated silicosis. In 1996, the International Agency for Research on Cancer (IARC) classified silica as carcinogenic to humans. There is evidence to suggest that silicosis patients have an increased risk of lung cancer, but it remains uncertain whether silica exposure alone increases lung cancer risk. Finally, there is the issue of airflow obstruction. Many of these patients smoke and have concomitant occupational dust exposure, as well as chronic bronchitis, all of which can lead to increased airflow obstruction over time.

Due to poor reporting and uncertain numbers of exposed individuals, information on the exact number of persons with silicosis is limited. In the United States between 1979 and 1990, there were 4,313 deaths attributed to silicosis as the primary or a contributing cause (2). Underreporting of the disease makes it likely that it is much more common, although it is difficult to know the true prevalence.

Asbestos has been used by humans for centuries for its qualities of fire resistance, tensile strength, and malleability. Asbestos is an industrial term that describes a variety of minerals (hydrated magnesium silicates) that break into fibers when crushed. The type of asbestos minerals (chrysotile, amosite, crocidolite, anthophyllite, tremolite, and actinolite) are important because they determine in part the disease potential. Industrialization increased the number of people exposed—although symptoms did not begin to develop until years after exposure. While it is well known to cause lung cancer and mesothelioma, asbestos also results in other diseases. Asbestosis is a scarring, or fibrotic lung, disease. The most common manifestation of asbestos-related disease is in the pleura. Pleural plaques are areas of thickened fibrous tissue, which often calcify. They cause no symptoms and may be found with other forms of asbestos-related disease. Fluid may collect in the pleural space (benign asbestos-related pleural effusion), which is believed to be a response to the pleural irritation by the asbestos fibers. The word "benign" is used to distinguish it from malignant mesothelioma, but the effusions can bring about chest discomfort and shortness of breath. These effusions may also be persistent and are a risk factor for pleural fibrosis.

Coal dust exposure can cause coal worker's pneumoconiosis (CWP), also known as black lung, which was recognized as a distinct entity from other pneumoconioses in the 1940s. Simple CWP is largely only an abnormality on the chest radiograph; there are small spots in the upper lung zones that reflect inhalation of coal dust, but nothing more. However, it can develop into complicated CWP, which is also called progressive massive fibrosis, a term and process shared with silicosis in which the smaller shadows coalesce into large nodules, 1 to 2 centimeters in diameter. These lesions can distort and destroy normal lung architecture and result in shortness of breath and disability. Exposure to coal dust has been found to result in airflow obstruction and chronic bronchitis and is also associated with the development of rheumatoid arthritis, which when combined with CWP is known as Caplan syndrome. Finally, an association of stomach cancer has been described in coal miners, potentially related to ingestion of the coal dust.

Other exposure-related diseases are "farmer's lung," or hypersensitivity pneumonitis (HP). Hypersensitivity pneumonitis, which was originally recognized by Bernardino Ramazzini in wheat reapers in 1713, is an interstitial lung disease caused by an immune response to an inhaled antigen. The well-described at-risk populations are farmers and bird hobbyists, but many other exposures can cause HP. The most recent addition is popcorn workers' lung, noted in workers and consumers with a history of heavy exposure to microwave popcorn butter flavoring. The true prevalence of HP is unknown because there

CASE STUDY

A 62-year-old man originally from Bolivia saw a physician for increasing shortness of breath. He had smoked one or two cigarettes a day for 15 years but quit at age 26. He immigrated to the United States at age 42 and worked for 12 months at a dental bridge manufacturing company, where he wore a mask while grinding bridges. At age 42, he was treated for suspicion of tuberculosis. Based on persistent abnormal chest x-ray images, he was diagnosed with accelerated silicosis with progressive massive fibrosis. A lung biopsy was performed to rule out lung cancer and showed mixed dust pneumoconiosis and silicosis, but no evidence of cancer. He was also found to have significant airflow obstruction and required oxygen supplementation. Currently, he is undergoing a lung transplant evaluation.

Comment

This case illustrates a number of points about silicosis. Many cases are arising from occupations not previously recognized as placing workers at risk. This lack of awareness means that these patients often are not diagnosed in a timely manner and continue to accrue exposure. Additionally, this case raises the issue of the elevated risk of tuberculosis and lung cancer in persons with silicosis. Because this patient came from a country with a high tuberculosis rate, it was likely he was exposed to the infection and at increased risk of developing active tuberculosis.

are many products that cause it; the illnesses have a great range of symptoms, and many people with mild disease do not seek medical attention. HP, however, has been reported to be present in as many as 12 percent of farmers and 20 percent of bird hobbyists (3).

Workers including sandblasters, miners, tunnelers, millers, and potters—among many others—are exposed to these inhaled particles and, therefore, are at risk of developing the disease. The true economic burden is difficult to estimate due to the uncertain number of at-risk individuals and likely underestimated prevalence numbers.

Table 1 Exposure, disease process, and prevalence of occupational lung diseases (1)

Occupational exposure	Disease	Prevalence in exposed population	Time of exposure to onset of symptoms
Silica	Acute Silicosis	Unknown	< 1 year
	Accelerated Silicosis	Unknown	3–10 years
	Chronic or Classic Silicosis	12.8 percent	Decades
Asbestos	Asbestosis	10–92 percent	Years
	Benign Asbestos Pleural Effusion	3 percent	< 20 years
	Pleural Plaques	6–70 percent	Years
Coal	Simple Coal Workers' Pneumoconiosis	5 percent	Years to decades
	Complicated Coal Workers' Pneumoconiosis (or Progressive Massive Fibrosis)	Unknown	Years to decades
Numerous (see Table 3)	Hypersensitivity Pneumonitis	12–20 percent	Day of exposure

Table 2 Occupational lung disease and its workforce exposure

Occupational lung disease	Exposed workforces
Silicosis	Sandblasters, miners, tunnelers, millers, potters, glassmakers, foundry and quarry workers, abrasive workers (including dental workers), silica flour mixers, and construction workers
Asbestos	Primary: Miners, millers Secondary: Asbestos insulators (laggers), ship building and repair, boilermakers, fireproofing, brake liners, ceramics workers Indirect: Electricians, plumbers, carpenters
Coal	Coal miners

What are we learning about the diseases?

Pathophysiology, causes: genetic, environment, microbes

In silicosis, fine (less than 5 micrometers) airborne particles of crystalline silica are inhaled and deposited in the smallest bronchioles and their neighboring alveoli. The disease-causing forms of silica are quartz, cristobalite, tridymite,

Table 3 Most frequent causes of hypersensitivity pneumonitis

Disease	Source of antigens
Plant products	
Farmer's lung	Moldy hay
Bagassosis	Moldy pressed sugarcane (bagasse)
Mushroom-worker's disease	Moldy compost
Malt-worker's lung	Contaminated barley
Maple bark disease	Contaminated maple logs
Sequoiosis	Contaminated wood dust
Wood pulp–worker's disease	Contaminated wood pulp
Humidifier lung	Contaminated humidifiers, air conditioners
Familial HP	Contaminated wood dust in walls
Compost lung	Compost
Cheese-washer's disease	Cheese casings
Wood-trimmer's disease	Contaminated wood trimmings
Thatched roof disease	Dried grasses and leaves
Tea-grower's disease	Tea plants
Coffee-worker's lung	Green coffee beans
Streptomyces albus HP	Contaminated fertilizer
Cephalosporium HP	Contaminated basement (sewage)
Sauna-taker's disease	Sauna water
Detergent-worker's disease	Detergent
Paprika-splitter's lung	Paprika dust
Japanese summer house HP	House dust; possibly bird droppings
Dry rot lung	Infected wood
Office-worker's or home HP	Dust from ventilation or heating systems

(continued on next page)

Occupational Lung Diseases

Disease	Source of antigens
Car air conditioner HP	Dust from air conditioner
Potato-riddler's lung	Moldy straw around potatoes
Tobacco-worker's disease	Mold on tobacco
Hot tub lung	Mycobacteria
Tap water lung	Contaminated water
Wine-grower's lung	Mold on grapes
Suberosis	Cork dust
Woodman's disease	Mold on bark
Saxophone lung	Saxophone mouthpiece
Grain-worker's lung	Grain dust
Fish meal–worker's lung	Fish meal dust
Soy sauce worker's HP	Fermenting soybeans

Animal products

Pigeon-breeder's disease	Pigeon droppings
Duck fever	Duck feathers
Turkey-handler's lung	Turkey products
Bird-fancier's lung	Bird products
Dove-pillow's lung	Bird feathers
Laboratory-worker's HP	Rat fur
Pituitary snuff–taker's disease	Pituitary powder
Mollusk shell HP	Mollusk shells

Insect products

Miller's lung	Wheat weevils

Reactive simple chemicals

TDI HP	Toluene diisocyanate

(continued on next page)

Disease	Source of antigens
TMA HP	Trimetallic anhydride
MDI HP	Diphenylmethane diisocyanate
Epoxy resin lung	Heated epoxy resin
Pauli's HP	Pauli's reagent
Popcorn worker's lung disease	Microwave popcorn flavoring

HP, hypersensitivity pneumonitis; IgA, immunoglobulin A; MDI, diphenylmethane diisocyanate; TDI, toluene diisocyanate; TMI, trimetallic anhydride.

and stishovite. Exactly how the damage occurs is not fully understood, but it is believed that freshly fractured particles of silica are the most dangerous, probably because the surface of the particles is more chemically active. These silica particles are taken up by the specialized cells (macrophages), which become activated and release oxidants, enzymes, growth factors, and other inflammatory mediators (cytokines). The macrophages eventually die and release the silica, which is indigestible. The silica particle is then taken up by other macrophages, and the process is perpetuated. As other inflammatory cells are recruited to the alveoli, the process continues to gather momentum, resulting in destruction of more cells and the tissue around them.

In the case of asbestos, the fibers are similarly inhaled, taken up by the macrophages and transported to the pleural space. The activated macrophages incite inflammation that can progress into fibrosis if the particles are not cleared. If the macrophages cannot eliminate the fibers, the needle-like particles are surrounded by an iron-containing protein (hemosiderin), forming what is called an "asbestos body." The extent of disease depends not only on the type of asbestos mineral but also on the intensity and duration of exposure.

In coal worker's pneumoconiosis, the disease begins with the inhalation of coal dust. Coal dust also is taken up by macrophages, which generate inflammatory cytokines and damaging oxidants. The spot on the chest radiograph is called a coal macule and consists of a collection of dust-laden macrophages surrounded by focal emphysema. Other factors that play a role in the degree of lung destruction are related to the coal. Intrinsic qualities of the coal have an

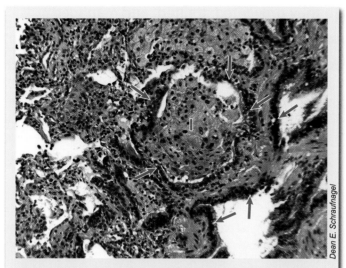

Inflammation in hypersensitivity pneumonitis is centered around the bronchi. The arrows in this microscopic view point to the bronchial lining cells. The small bronchioles are often plugged with inflammatory cells (I). Collections of cells called granulomas are often present but not shown here.

impact on disease—the higher the carbon content, the higher the risk of disease. With the exception of drillers, surface coal miners tend to have less CWP. The level of silica exposure during the mining process can dictate who develops silicosis; the lung disease caused by silica and coal exposure can be difficult to distinguish from each other clinically.

Hypersensitivity pneumonitis is an allergic reaction. The first step involves exposure to an antigen of organic material from bacterial, fungal, plant, or animal proteins. Initial exposure results in sensitization in which the body forms antibodies to these antigens. Repeated exposure results in inflammation. If the exposure is not halted, it can permanently damage the lung. Due to this, HP represents a continuum of disease sometimes categorized as acute, subacute, and chronic. It is likely that some individuals may have a genetic predisposition to HP. Interestingly, the damage that smoking causes may decrease the delivery of the antigen to the alveoli and decrease the antibody response, resulting in a lower risk of HP.

How are they prevented, treated, and managed?

Prevention, treatment, staying healthy, prognosis

For asbestos, coal, and silica-related disease, there is no treatment other than optimizing the patient's current health and preventing further exposure. Prognosis varies depending on the severity of the disease. Persons with simple CWP or classic silicosis may never experience symptoms, whereas complicated CWP results in severe respiratory debilitation and death. Although these materials are present in nature, it is their mining and commercial use that generates the toxic exposure for humans.

Worldwide production of asbestos peaked in the 1970s, but there were still over 2 million tons of asbestos mined in 2000 (4). In 2005, the Collegium Ramazzini, an international organization of occupational and environmental scientists, called for a worldwide ban on commercial use of asbestos, but it is estimated that worldwide 125 million people still are exposed to asbestos in the workplace, and 90,000 people die each year from lung cancer, malignant mesothelioma, and asbestosis secondary to asbestos exposure. Moreover, since the use of asbestos has been banned in the United States only since the 1990s, the peak of disease incidence may lie ahead. The prognosis for mesothelioma and lung cancer is dismal, with less than 20 percent 5-year survival rates. For all individuals exposed to asbestos, there is the need for surveillance for development of malignancy.

Coal is only used as a fuel and, therefore, exposure is limited to miners. Aggressive regulations in the coal industry have resulted in reductions in the burden of disease. In 1969, the Federal Coal Mine Health and Safety Act was passed, which put in place standards designed to ensure that cumulative exposure over the typical career span of 25 years would not exceed levels known to cause respiratory impairment. Effective in 1980, the respirable coal mine dust standard was decreased from 3 to 2 milligrams per cubic meter (mg/m^3). These regulations have served to decrease the prevalence rate of CWP among 25-year mine workers from 20 percent in 1987 to slightly more than 5 percent in 2002 (1). In conjunction with these standards, secondary prevention measures also require all coal miners to receive regular medical screening. Furthermore, if a worker shows signs of CWP, he or she has the option of transferring to a lower-dust area (less than 1 mg/m^3) and receiving increased monitoring. All patients are encouraged to stop smoking, and other treatments are offered as clinically indicated.

Silica is the least regulated of the agents causing occupational lung diseases. Silicosis is an irreversible fibrotic process without a cure. Treatment rests on preventing further insult to the lungs. Reduction in risk of tuberculosis is also critically important, and all patients should be screened for latent or active tuberculosis infection and evaluated for other tuberculosis risk factors, such as HIV infection. As with any lung disease, smoking cessation is a must. In treatment trials thus far, no drug has been found to halt the progression of disease.

In the case of hypersensitivity pneumonitis, treatment consists of removing the source of the exposure and eradicating any residual antigens to prevent re-exposure—for example, drying hay to prevent molding or removing stagnant water to prevent bacterial or fungal overgrowth. Often, the most challenging part of care is convincing the patient that removal of the antigen is necessary or that he or she must leave the workplace. If the disease is severe at diagnosis, a short course of oral corticosteroids can help expedite recovery. The prognosis depends on the degree of continued exposure. Farmers are often exposed at the end of winter when using the remainder of the previous year's hay supply. Because this exposure is usually self-limited and occurs once a year, most individuals will recover completely. Conversely, the individual who has repeated or long-term exposure might suffer permanent damage to the lungs.

Are we making a difference?

Research past, present, and future

Each of the occupational diseases begins with the inhalation of disease-inducing particles. Therefore, the main goals have been to identify and regulate the industries that generate these particles on one hand and to determine ways to prevent or minimize their inhalation on the other. In dealing with silica, coal, and asbestos, the significant latency period between exposure and diagnosis makes it difficult to determine dose–response relationships.

There is no treatment for any of the occupational diseases that can reverse the damage already done. However, for those who were or continue to be exposed, the search for treatments must continue. Early reports of gene therapy resulting in anti-tumor responses may hold promise for those with mesothelioma. Research in pulmonary fibrosis may be applicable to asbestosis in the future. In the case of HP, early research was based on observation and the discovery of the causative antigens, the removal of which improved symptoms. Studying the patient's serum allowed the discovery of antibodies that reacted with the specific antigen (precipitins). It is still not possible to predict who will develop HP, which antigens set up the inflammation, and how or in whom the disease will progress, but there are reasons to hope. Certain genetic predispositions have been discovered, and recent studies in the mouse have shown that certain cells and their signaling cytokines are important in the pathogenesis of HP.

What we need to cure or eliminate occupational lung diseases

In occupational lung diseases, the primary strategy must be prevention. Strong federal regulations and funding for CWP prevention in conjunction with scientific research have laid a foundation for a continuing reduction of the burden of disease in the United States. This approach should serve as a model for how to proceed in preventing other occupational lung diseases.

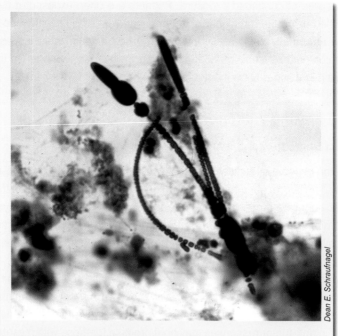

Dean E. Schraufnagel

Needle-like asbestos particles penetrate the lung and cannot be dissolved or destroyed by the body. Instead, the body coats them with a protein associated with iron. The presence of asbestos bodies in the lungs only signifies exposure, not disease.

When the underlying disease mechanism is understood, as it is with smallpox and polio, there is the potential to eliminate the disease. In the case of asbestos-related diseases, the etiology is known—without asbestos exposure there is no asbestos-related disease. A worldwide ban of asbestos would eventually virtually eliminate its associated diseases.

Increased monitoring of air concentrations of silica in the workplace, as well as duration of exposure for workers, is necessary. A registry that then follows populations of workers over time to determine the rate of silicosis would help to determine if there are safe levels of silica exposure in the workplace. Based on this, regulations could be enacted worldwide to decrease the burden of silicosis. For those who are unfortunate enough to develop silicosis, continued research on the pathogenesis of the disease and studies on whether or not there is a genetic component could help develop potential treatments.

In the case of HP, increased awareness in the community and in relevant industries will help to bring patients to medical attention earlier in their disease process. More organized follow-up will help to better characterize the natural history of the disease and cease exposure. An organized reporting system for new cases would serve to initiate the proper investigation in a timely fashion. Further research on signaling cytokines could lead to new treatment or preventative options.

References

1. Rom WN, Markowitz S, eds. *Environmental and Occupational Medicine*. 4th ed. Philadelphia, PA: Lippincott Williams & Wilkins; 2007.
2. Adverse effects of crystalline silica exposure. American Thoracic Society Committee of the Scientific Assembly on Environmental and Occupational Health. *Am J Respir Crit Care Med* 1997;155:761–768.
3. Mason RJ, Murray JF, Nadel JA, Broaddus VC, eds. *Murray and Nadel's Textbook of Respiratory Medicine*. 4th ed. Philadelphia, PA: Elsevier Saunders; 2005.
4. World Health Organization. *Elimination of Asbestos-Related Diseases*. Geneva, Switzerland: World Health Organization; 2006.

Web sites of interest

International Agency for Research on Cancer
www.iarc.fr

World Health Organization
www.who.int/en/

14

Pleural Disease

The pleura is a thin tissue covered by a layer of cells (mesothelial cells) that surrounds the lungs and lines the inside of the chest wall. The pleural space is the area between the lungs and the chest wall. It is normally at subatmospheric pressure, which keeps the lungs inflated. The normal pleural space has only a few milliliters of liquid, which helps lubricate the normal to and fro motion of the lungs during breathing. Fluid, air, and particles can move into the pleural space from different parts of the body because of its low pressure and its ability to hold large amounts of liquid or air. Pleural effusion (large amounts of liquid in the pleural space) or pneumothorax (air in the pleural space) can lead to a partial or complete compression of the lung.

If a tear or hole develops in the lung, air escapes into the pleural space, causing a pneumothorax. Sometimes, air goes into the pleural space and is trapped there under high pressure, causing a "tension pneumothorax" that can stop blood from returning to the heart and lead to death if not recognized and treated promptly. In addition, inhaled toxic particles such as asbestos can move into the pleural space where, decades later, mesothelioma can develop.

Whom does it affect?

Epidemiology, prevalence, economic burden, vulnerable populations

Many diseases affect the pleural space in both adults and children, including common diseases such as pneumonia, breast cancer, and heart failure. Pleural disease is, therefore, often a secondary effect of another disease process. Pleural effusion is the most common manifestation of pleural disease and a common presentation of other conditions such as heart failure or kidney failure. It is estimated that a million Americans develop a pleural effusion each year (1). "Pleurisy" is any inflammatory condition of the pleura. Because the pleura is richly supplied with nerves, pleurisy can be quite painful. Usually, when the pleural space is involved in pneumonia or lung cancer, the patient is sicker and has a worse prognosis than in the absence of pleural involvement.

A common cause of pleural disease is cancer. It is estimated that malignant pleural effusion affects 150,000 people per year in the United States (2). Most patients with pleural effusion come to the doctor complaining of shortness of breath, which is caused by fluid accumulating in the chest and compressing the lung (2). Once a malignant pleural effusion is diagnosed, the prognosis is very poor, with patients living only another four months on average.

Approximate annual incidence of various types of pleural effusions in adults in the United States

Type	Incidence
Congestive heart failure	500,000
Parapneumonic effusion	300,000
Malignant pleural effusion	200,000
Pulmonary embolism	150,000
Viral disease	100,000
Post–coronary artery bypass	50,000
Gastrointestinal disease	25,000
Tuberculosis	2,500
Mesothelioma	2,704
Asbestos exposure	2,000

Adapted from (5).

CASE STUDY

In 1979, film icon Steve McQueen was diagnosed with mesothelioma at age 49, after complaining to his doctor of chronic cough and shortness of breath with exertion. He was told the cause of the disease was his exposure to asbestos as a young man working in construction and as a merchant marine. Asbestos insulation was used extensively in ships at that time, and he recalled occasions when the air was clouded with asbestos dust as he cleaned a ship's engine room after pipe installation.

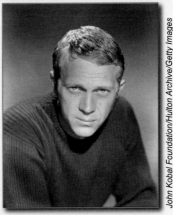

John Kobal Foundation/Hulton Archive/Getty Images

After being told that his condition was terminal and that he had less than a year to live, McQueen sought help from a clinic in Mexico that claimed miraculous cures. He underwent a regimen involving animal cell injections, coffee enemas, Laetrile, and huge daily doses of vitamin pills. But his health only worsened, and the tumors in his chest and abdomen continued to grow, causing him pain and shortness of breath. In a final attempt to extend his life and reduce his discomfort, he underwent an operation in Mexico to remove a tumor from his abdomen, but died shortly afterward.

Comment

At the time of his diagnosis, there was no treatment for mesothelioma, a cancer that progressively reduces a person's ability to breathe and can cause considerable pain. Although the public accounts of McQueen's illness do not mention chest pain, this symptom is a nearly universal complaint among those with mesothelioma. Unfortunately, more than 30 years later, the prognosis for malignant mesothelioma is not much different than it was in McQueen's time. The McQueen story of a desperate attempt to find a cure continues to challenge science and medicine today.

Persons involved in automobile accidents or any trauma are also at increased risk for pneumothorax. Pleural fibrosis and lung compression can follow pleural infection or injury. The primary pleural cancer, mesothelioma, is a risk for anyone exposed to asbestos. Asbestos continues to be used in certain U.S. industries and is found in many buildings. Disruption of these buildings can expose persons to asbestos (2). The World Trade Center collapse introduced tons of asbestos into the environment, and it is believed that there will be an increased risk of mesothelioma among those who worked at the site (3). However, because mesothelioma develops an average of 35 to 40 years after the time of exposure, these cases are not expected to be identified until approximately 2036. Unfortunately, there is no effective screening tool for early detection of this disease.

An uncommon disease that affects the pleural space is lymphangioleiomyomatosis (LAM). This disorder almost exclusively affects women of reproductive age and is characterized by abnormal growth of smooth-muscle cells around the small airways and small blood and lymph vessels of the lung. The pleural space involvement is a major issue for these patients. As of June 2009, there were 1,247 living patients in the database of the LAM Foundation. Of these, 483 persons had suffered a pneumothorax, 187 had a pleural effusion, and 24 developed a very unusual pleural effusion caused by a rupture of a lymphatic channel that spills essential dietary fats into the pleural space (chylous pleural effusion). Patients with LAM have the highest rate of pneumothorax of all chronic lung diseases (60 to 70 percent); the recurrence rate is 66 percent without treatment (4).

The economic burden of pleural disease is difficult to estimate, but it is undoubtedly enormous, given the number of diseases with which the pleura is involved and the frequent need for hospitalization and surgery to treat pleural involvement.

What are we learning about this disease?

Pathophysiology, causes: genetic, environment, microbes

A great deal has been learned about the diseases that involve the pleural space. These diseases often reflect diseases elsewhere in the body that spread to the pleural space, whether the process is infection, inflammation, cancer, or edema. The fluid movement into and out of the pleural space is governed by pressure

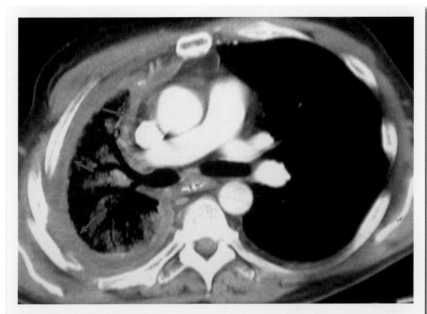

In this CT scan, mesothelioma is shown growing extensively in the pleural space (arrows) and is completely surrounding the lung on one side of the chest. The thickened pleura can be appreciated in comparison to the same area on the opposite side, which is normal. Note how the chest on the side of the mesothelioma is smaller than the opposite side; mesothelioma characteristically shrinks the chest and constricts the lung, making it difficult to take a breath. One can also appreciate how difficult it would be to treat a tumor that spreads in this way (2).

differences that arise from breathing and blood flow, but there are many active cellular processes that keep excessive fluid out of the normal pleural space. There are genetic, environmental, and infectious causes of diseases that spread to the pleura, and certain ones affect the pleura more than the rest of the lung.

Mesothelioma, the cancer of mesothelial cells suffered by Steve McQueen, is caused by inhalation of asbestos fibers, which commonly cause other disorders of the pleura as well, including chronic pleural effusions and benign tumors. Tuberculosis and certain other infections also commonly affect the pleura. Some disease processes do not generally affect the pleura, and this feature is useful in diagnosis. For example, collagen vascular diseases (see Chapter 6) often involve the pleura, while most interstitial lung diseases do not. Other genetic and environmental factors have lesser effects on pleural disease.

Deaths due to mesothelioma in the United States

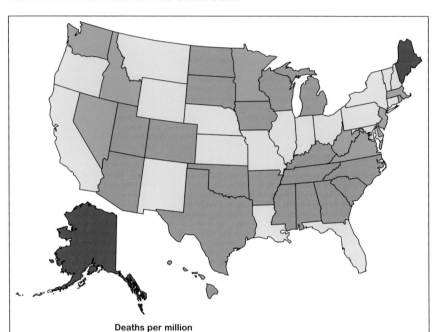

Deaths per million
■ >20.0   ■ 15.1–20.0   □ 10.1–15.0   ■ <10.1

The geographical location of mesothelioma is not randomly distributed and may reflect differences in asbestos use. From NIOSH publication No. 2004-146, Worker Health Chartbook 2004.

How is it prevented, treated, and managed?

Prevention, treatment, staying healthy, prognosis

Because pleural disease has many causes and frequently results from disease centered elsewhere in the body, there is no universal way to prevent it. However, some causes of pleural disease, such as tuberculosis and asbestos exposure, are preventable.

The pleural space may be the first site where a disease manifests itself, providing the diagnosis of a distant problem. The diagnosis is usually made by sampling the liquid in the pleural space to analyze the cells and proteins and to test for bacteria, cancer cells, or other disease markers.

Liquid or air in the pleural space can be removed by sterile tubes placed into it through the chest wall. Placement of this type of tube can also be performed

Percent of cases with pleural disease for various conditions in adults in the United States

Disease	Percent with pleural involvement
Bacterial pneumonia	44%
Lupus	93% (disease at autopsy)
	45–60% (inflammation of pleura)
Rheumatoid arthritis	20%
Systemic sclerosis—diffuse	10%
Sarcoidosis	2.8%
Wegener's granulomatosis	<10%
End-stage renal disease	2–16%
Pulmonary embolism	48%
Post–cardiac injury	10% (large fluid collection)
Lymphangioleiomyomatosis	60–81% (pneumothorax)
	22–39% (chylothorax)

Adapted from (5).

Percent of cases with pleural disease for various conditions in children in the United States

Type	Incidence
Bacterial pneumonia/hospitalized	40%
Tuberculosis	5%
Lupus	33%
Post–cardiac surgery	0.9–4.7% (chylothorax)

Adapted from (5).

emergently when there is a tension pneumothorax. However, in the case of pleural effusions, removal of liquid must be carefully calibrated. If too much fluid is removed too quickly, the lung can be injured by rapid re-expansion. Infection can add another complication. If the pleural space is infected, the inflammation can cause the two pleural layers to adhere to each other, which then could separate the fluid into small pockets that cannot be removed easily. Cancer may also grow through both pleural layers and fix them together, thus preventing full lung expansion. Removal of infected fluid can sometimes be improved by injecting certain enzymes into the pleural space that break down the fibrous material that causes the pleural layers to stick together.

Once the pleural space is emptied of its fluid or air, the next therapy is often to obliterate the space to prevent fluid from returning and compromising breathing. The procedure is called *pleurodesis* and is performed on as many as 100,000 patients per year in the United States to treat recurrent pleural effusions (1). The technique usually involves injection into the pleural space of an irritating agent, such as talc. However, talc pleurodesis is only 60 to 80 percent effective and may itself be injurious, depending on the qualities of the talc used. Previously, as many as 9 percent of those receiving talc went on to develop a lung injury (6), but it is now thought that this complication may be avoided if larger particles of talc are used.

There are no specific measures that patients should adopt to maintain "healthy" pleura other than to avoid exposure to environmental toxins known to cause pleural diseases, such as asbestos fibers. The prognosis of pleural diseases depends on the underlying cause and ranges from very poor (for example, when cancer has spread to the pleura) to very good (for example, when an otherwise healthy person develops fluid associated with a treatable infection).

Are we making a difference?

Research past, present, and future

A number of advances have been made in understanding the physiology of the pleura and the pleural space, but exactly how and why the pleural cavity is affected by certain diseases but not others is largely unknown. Other mysteries also remain, such as why it takes so long for mesothelioma to develop after the initial asbestos exposure.

However, new diagnostic advances, including blood and pleural fluid tests, can assist with diagnosis in difficult settings. New imaging advances, such as bedside ultrasound and positron emission tomography (PET) scans, have helped foster a better medical understanding of the anatomy and function of the pleural tissues. Video-assisted thoracoscopy surgery (VATS) offers a minimally invasive method for doctors to view and biopsy the pleura and its contents.

Already, recently developed tests of the pleural fluid have allowed diagnoses to be made without the need for invasive biopsies. Biological assays, such as N-terminal pro–brain natriuretic peptide, have improved the diagnosis of pleural effusion caused by heart failure. Microarray chips that can detect the presence of up to thousands of genes at a single time show great promise in testing the genetics of cancer cells and helping to diagnose and guide treatment. For example, discovery of certain mutations (such as epidermal growth factor receptor (EGFR) in cancer cells of pleural effusions has allowed selection of cancer therapies that inhibit the relevant molecular pathway and may improve responses.

However, an early-screening test for mesothelioma remains out of reach. Researchers are now working on developing blood, pleural fluid, and even breath tests that may be able to detect chemical substances that are produced uniquely by a specific tumor or infecting organism or are produced by the body in response to asbestos.

Although progress is being made in the diagnosis of pleural disease, treatment lags behind that of other respiratory conditions. Talc was first used in 1935 by Dr. Norman Bethune, a noted thoracic surgeon. Despite its limited effectiveness, little advancement has been made in this area. Treatment approaches are being studied that could lead to more effective and less invasive ways of caring for patients with pleural disease. Newer tubes and reservoirs for patients with chronic pleural disease have reduced the need to remain in the hospital. Agents that induce an effective, quick, and painless pleurodesis could greatly improve patient care by speeding and simplifying the process and reducing the complications of lung injury and pleural scarring. Better agents to break down fibrin might also prevent the need for surgery. Other ways to attack pleural disease, such as by controlling the inflammatory response or targeting the tumor cells (6), hold promise. Agents that are injected directly into the pleural cavity have the additional advantage of reducing toxicity to other organs.

It is not possible to think in terms of cure for pleural disease because it is often a disease that originates outside the pleura and has many etiologies. Although mesothelioma should eventually decrease as asbestos is replaced, "cure" for pleural disease awaits cures of other conditions.

References

1. Lee YCG, Light RW. Future directions. In: Light RW, Lee YCG, eds. *Textbook of Pleural Diseases*. London, England: Hodder Arnold; 2003:536–541.
2. Boylan A, Broaddus VC. Tumors of the pleura. In: Mason RJ, Murray JF, Nadel JA, Broaddus VC, eds. *Murray and Nadel's Textbook of Respiratory Medicine*. 4th ed. Philadelphia, PA: Elsevier Health Sciences; 2005:1989–2010.
3. Landrigan PJ, Lioy PH, Thurston G, Berkowitz G, Chen LC, Chillrud SN, Gavett SH, Georgopoulos PG, Geyh AS, Levin S, et al. Health and environmental consequences of the world trade center disaster. *Environ Health Perspect* 2004;112:731–739.
4. Almoosa KF, McCormack FX, Sahn SA. Pleural disease in lymphangioleiomyomatosis. *Clin Chest Med* 2006;27:355–368
5. Light RW. *Pleural Diseases*. 5th ed. Philadelphia, PA: Lippincott Williams & Wilkins; 2007.
6. Heffner JE, Klein JS. Recent advances in the diagnosis and management of malignant pleural effusions. *Mayo Clin Proc* 2008;83:235–250

Web sites of interest

The British Thoracic Society
www.brit-thoracic.org.uk

International Pleural Newsletter
www.musc.edu/pleuralnews/IPN

International Mesothelioma Interest Group
www.imig.org

The LAM Foundation
www.thelamfoundation.org

NIOSH: National Institute for Occupational Safety and Health
Occupational Respiratory Disease Surveillance National Statistics
webappa.cdc.gov/ords/norms-icd.html

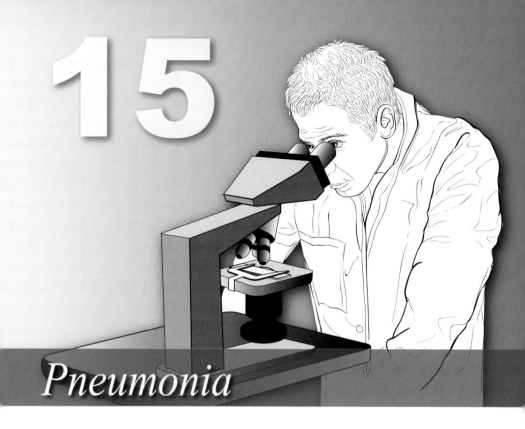

15

Pneumonia

Pneumonia is a lung infection involving the lung alveoli (air sacs) and can be caused by microbes, including bacteria, viruses, or fungi. It is the leading infectious cause of hospitalization and death in the United States and exacts an enormous cost in economic and human terms. Healthy individuals can develop pneumonia, but susceptibility is greatly increased by a variety of personal characteristics.

Whom does it affect?

Epidemiology, prevalence, economic burden, vulnerable populations

Pneumonia was described 2,500 years ago by Hippocrates, the father of medicine. Dr. William Osler, the founder of modern medicine, who studied pneumonia throughout his career, called pneumonia the "captain of the men of death" because of the great toll it exacted on humanity. Pneumonia occurs commonly in individuals living in their home communities ("community-acquired pneumonia") as well as in individuals who are hospitalized for other reasons ("hospital-acquired pneumonia"). In the 1930s, before the advent of antibiotics, pneumonia was the third-leading cause of death in the United States. Notably, it remains a leading cause of death. In 2006, it was the eighth-leading cause of death,

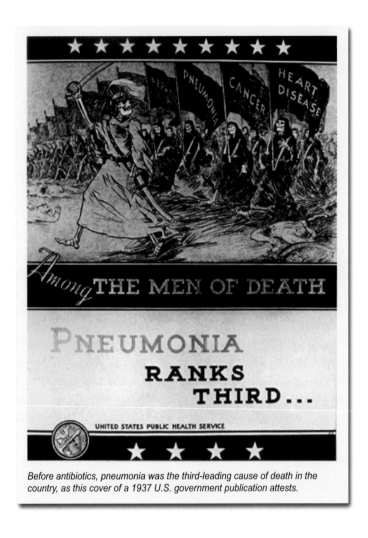

★ ★ ★ ★ ★ ★ ★ ★ ★ ★

Among THE MEN OF DEATH

PNEUMONIA
RANKS
THIRD...

UNITED STATES PUBLIC HEALTH SERVICE

★ ★ ★ ★

Before antibiotics, pneumonia was the third-leading cause of death in the country, as this cover of a 1937 U.S. government publication attests.

accounting for about 55,000 deaths (1). It is estimated that 4 million cases of community-acquired pneumonia occur annually in the United States, of which 20 to 25 percent are severe enough to warrant hospitalization. Pneumonia is second only to delivering a baby as a cause for hospitalization in the United States today (1).

The human and economic burden of pneumonia is enormous. In fact, World Health Organization data indicate that respiratory infections, a term which in this

Pneumonia is the leading killer of children under the age of five worldwide

	% total under-five deaths	Region
21%	13%	South Asia
21%	7%	Sub-Saharan Africa
15%	11%	Middle East and North Africa
15%	9%	East Asia and Pacific
14%	8%	Latin America and Caribbean
13%	8%	CEE/CIS (Central and Eastern Europe and the Commonwealth of Independent States)
20%	9%	Developing Countries
2% 3%		Industrialized world
19%	10%	World

0   20   40   60   80   100

% total under-five deaths

■ Pneumonia   ■ Neonatal severe infections (mainly pneumonia/sepsis)

This bar chart shows that pneumonia is the leading killer of children under five worldwide. "Pneumonia: The forgotten killer of children," The United Nations Children's Fund (UNICEF)/World Health Organization (WHO), 2006.

context is synonymous with pneumonia, account for more deaths among children worldwide than any other cause and for more disability-adjusted life years lost around the world than any other category of disease, including cancer and cardiovascular disease (2). In the United States alone, total medical expenditures and indirect costs (lost work and productivity) attributed to pneumonia amounted to more than $40 billion in 2005 (1).

The lungs are particularly susceptible to infection because they interact with the outside environment. They are exposed to about 10,000 liters of air per day, which may contain infectious or toxic agents. The lungs are also connected to the upper airways and are, therefore, frequently exposed to small amounts of saliva and oral secretions that contain bacteria. Furthermore, part of the passageway to the lungs is shared by the stomach, and stomach contents can, on occasion, be regurgitated and aspirated into the lungs.

Although pneumonia can occur in anyone, it occurs with increased frequency in individuals whose immune systems are deficient (3). Human

CASE STUDY

An 85-year-old woman with a history of COPD associated with past smoking complained of fatigue along with increased shortness of breath and white-grey sputum. She had no fever or chest pain. When she arrived at the hospital, she had low blood pressure, low blood oxygen levels, an elevated white blood cell count, and a new shadow on the chest x-ray image of her right lung, which confirmed the diagnosis of pneumonia. She was admitted to the intensive care unit with a diagnosis of community-acquired pneumonia and possible sepsis. (Sepsis is the term used to indicate that the infection has spread throughout the body via the bloodstream.) She was treated with intravenous antibiotics, fluids, blood pressure support medications, and oxygen via a face mask. She improved, but because of a persistent high oxygen requirement, she underwent a computed tomography (CT) scan that revealed a large fluid collection around her right lung. Two needle drainage procedures of this fluid ultimately resulted in improvement in her shortness of breath and her oxygen requirement. She returned home after two weeks in the hospital. No bacteria were ever identified in cultures of her sputum, blood, or fluid around the lung.

Comment

This patient was vulnerable to pneumonia because of her age and her underlying COPD. As in many elderly persons, her pneumonia presented with vague symptoms such as fatigue and confusion. Her lack of fever, which can be seen with pneumonia, reflects an inadequate immune response to the infection and, again, was likely owing to her age. She illustrates serious and common complications of pneumonia. She had a sepsis-like picture with an overwhelming reaction that caused a fall in blood pressure (shock). Sepsis and respiratory failure are major causes of death in pneumonia patients. Fluid collection around the lung (pleural effusion) and low oxygen levels are other common complications. The lack of identified bacteria in cultures of pneumonia patients' blood is common, as bacteria may not be present in the blood at the precise moment when the cultures are drawn, or their growth may be suppressed by prior administration of antibiotics.

immunodeficiency virus (HIV) infection, malnutrition, diabetes, renal failure, cancers, and treatment with immunosuppressive drugs are all risk factors for developing pneumonia. Infants and very young children are highly vulnerable, as are the elderly. At both extremes of age, this increased risk relates in part to impaired immunity. In the United States, individuals older than age 65 account for almost two thirds of hospitalizations and 90 percent of deaths from pneumonia (4).

Patients who smoke or have underlying lung diseases, including chronic obstructive pulmonary disease (COPD), cystic fibrosis, congestive heart failure, and lung cancer, are also vulnerable, owing to abnormalities in lung structure and function. Finally, patients with respiratory failure who are on mechanical ventilators are more prone to pneumonia (3).

What are we learning about this disease?

Pathophysiology, causes: genetic, environment, microbes

Pneumonia can be transmitted when airborne microbes from an infected individual are inhaled by someone else. However, most instances of pneumonia are attributable to self-infection with one or more types of microbes that originate in the nose and mouth. In healthy people, typical upper airway bacterial residents such as *Streptococcus pneumoniae* (commonly referred to as "pneumococcus") and *Hemophilus influenzae* are the most common bacteria causing community-acquired pneumonia. Hospital-acquired pneumonia is usually caused by more resistant bacteria, such as *Staphylococcus aureus, Klebsiella pneumoniae, Pseudomonas aeruginosa,* and *Escherichia coli.* Individuals with a serious impairment of their immune system become susceptible to pneumonia caused by so-called "opportunistic" microbes, such as certain fungi, viruses, and bacteria related to tuberculosis (mycobacteria), that would not ordinarily cause disease in normal individuals (5).

To cope with its constant exposure to potentially infectious microbes, the lung depends on a hierarchy of defense mechanisms (3). Physical mechanisms that can prevent microbes from reaching the alveoli include the structure of the upper airway, the branching of the bronchial tree, the sticky mucus layer lining the airways, the hair-like cilia that propel mucus upward, and the cough reflex. The microbes that do manage to reach the alveoli are usually destroyed by a variety of immune cells, which is why most pneumonias occur in people with one or more deficiencies in either their mechanical or immune defense mechanisms.

How is it prevented, treated, and managed?

Prevention, treatment, staying healthy, prognosis

Although pneumonia cannot be completely prevented, a variety of strategies can be employed to reduce its incidence. Adequate nutrition, dental hygiene, and not smoking are elements of a healthy lifestyle that reduce a person's risk of getting pneumonia.

For those with lung disease or impaired clearance of mucus, aerobic exercise, deep breathing maneuvers, and cough assist devices can facilitate expectoration and lung hygiene. Immunity to certain common microbes can also be enhanced by immunization of vulnerable populations with specific vaccines. In contrast to the influenza vaccine, which must be administered annually to keep up with the ever-changing strains of influenza virus, the vaccine against *Streptococcus pneumoniae* bacteria typically provides longer-term protection.

Pneumonia is generally diagnosed based on a history of typical symptoms, abnormal breath sounds that can be heard with a stethoscope, a chest radiograph showing characteristic shadows, and, sometimes, laboratory tests (5). Once the disease is recognized, a determination is made as to its severity and whether the patient requires hospitalization. Approximately 75 percent of cases are managed as outpatients with oral antibiotics and fluids; this manifestation is sometimes called "walking pneumonia."

Since the responsible microbe is usually not known initially (and is often never definitively identified), antibacterial agents are selected to cover the most likely culprits. Many viral causes of pneumonia lack effective drug treatments, but fortunately, most healthy patients will recover from either bacterial or viral pneumonia with no long-term consequences.

As the population has aged and as the number of patients with multiple vulnerabilities has increased, the proportion requiring hospitalization for pneumonia and experiencing poor outcomes has grown. Also contributing to adverse outcomes is the growing problem of microbes that are resistant to antibiotics to which they were formerly sensitive. An important factor driving antibiotic resistance has been the inappropriate use of antibiotics when they are not called for, such as for the common cold.

Are we making a difference?

Research past, present, and future

In almost no area of medicine has a discovery made a greater impact than that of antibiotics for infections. The availability of penicillin starting in the 1940s revolutionized the treatment of patients with pneumococcal pneumonia, which previously had been limited to watchful waiting. This discovery laid the ground-work for the development of additional antibiotics for treatment of other bacterial, viral, and fungal forms of pneumonia. In recent years, research on vaccinations has increased and has already reduced the frequency of the most common forms of pneumonia. The means to diagnose pneumonia have improved with better sampling procedures, such as bronchoscopy, and new methods for rapid laboratory detection of microbial molecules in sputum, blood, and urine.

Global burden of disease (DALYs lost in 2002, worldwide)

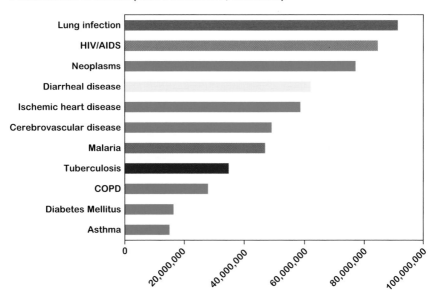

Pneumonia causes the greatest burden of any disease when measured by disability-adjusted life years (DALYs) lost. World Health Organization 2002 (3).

Despite these major advances, the dimensions of the clinical problem posed by pneumonia remain enormous. After those early gains achieved with first-generation antibiotics, the mortality rate for pneumonia has not changed appreciably in the last 50 years (6).

What we need to cure or eliminate pneumonia

In order to take the next leap forward to reduce the burden of pneumonia, the following issues must be tackled: 1) new laboratory approaches must be developed that are capable of rapidly identifying the causative microbe so that physicians can more precisely select antimicrobial drugs for treatment of pneumonia; 2) effective antibiotics must be developed against microbes for which there are currently none available; and 3) existing vaccines need to be improved and new vaccines developed.

However, vaccines cannot be developed against every microbe. Old microbes continuously change and new ones emerge. New antibiotics alone will not be enough because microbes develop antibiotic resistance. A substantial investigative effort must be mounted to improve the understanding of lung immunity—how it functions to deal with various infections, how it is influenced by common host factors, and how it can be manipulated for therapeutic gain. To complement antibiotics, an array of immunostimulant strategies that can be intelligently applied in different types of patients is needed. Substances that stimulate immunity could also be employed to enhance the body's response to vaccination.

References

1. Centers for Disease Control and Prevention Web site. Pneumonia. Available at: http://www.cdc.gov/nchs/FASTATS/pneumonia.htm. Accessed February 6, 2010.
2. Mizgerd JP. Lung infection—a public health priority. *PLoS Med* 2006;3:e76.
3. Mizgerd JP. Acute lower respiratory tract infection. *N Engl J Med* 2008;358:716–727.
4. Fry AM, Shay DK, Holman RC, Curns AT, Anderson LJ. Trends in hospitalizations for pneumonia among persons aged 65 years or older in the United States, 1988–2002. *JAMA* 2005;294:2712–2719.
5. Medline Plus Web site. Pneumonia. Available at: http://www.nlm.nih.gov/medlineplus/ency/article/000145.htm. Accessed February 6, 2010.
6. Wunderink RG, Mutlu GM. Pneumonia: overview and epidemiology. In: Laurent GJ, Shapiro SD, eds. *Encyclopedia of Respiratory Medicine*. Oxford, UK: Elsevier Academic Press; 2006:402–410.

Web sites of interest

Medline Plus
Pneumonia
www.nlm.nih.gov/medlineplus/ency/article/000145.htm

Centers for Disease Control and Prevention
Pneumonia
www.cdc.gov/nchs/FASTATS/pneumonia.htm

American Thoracic Society
Infectious Diseases Society of America/American Thoracic Society Consensus Guidelines on Managing Community-Acquired Pneumonia
www.thoracic.org/statements/resources/mtpi/idsaats-cap.pdf

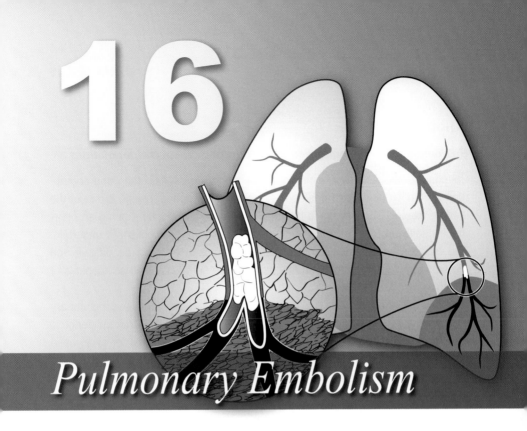

Pulmonary Embolism

If blood flowing within the blood vessels of the body stops, the tissue it supplies could die from lack of oxygen. If, after a serious wound, blood flowing outside the body does not stop, a person could die from hemorrhage. Yet, the blood within the blood vessels flows almost perfectly throughout life, and bleeding usually stops within minutes after a cut. Occasionally, blood can clot within the blood vessels, which is called a *thrombus*. Abnormal material floating in the blood is called an *embolus*. A thrombus that breaks free and floats in the moving bloodstream is called a *thromboembolism*. The blood in the veins, with its slow flow and low pressure, is more likely to clot (*venous thrombus*) than blood in the arteries; it may go to the lungs (*pulmonary embolism* or *venous thromboembolism*), where it can become lodged in the small blood vessels. An embolism can also be caused by other material floating free in the bloodstream, as in, for example, tumor embolism or foreign-body embolism, but these conditions are rare compared to thromboemboli and are not considered further in this chapter.

Blood coagulation is highly regulated; a moving stream works to prevent clotting, and stagnant blood promotes clotting. Tissue injury triggers blood clotting, and any defect in the many factors controlling clotting may increase or decrease the chance of blood coagulation.

Pulmonary emboli are common, difficult to diagnose, and often deadly.

Whom does it affect?

Epidemiology, prevalence, economic burden, vulnerable populations

Pulmonary embolism is a common complication of hospitalization and contributes to 5 to 10 percent of deaths in hospitalized patients, making it one of the leading causes of preventable hospital deaths (1–4). Despite it being an enormous health problem, the true incidence of pulmonary embolism is uncertain. The diagnosis of venous thrombi and pulmonary emboli can be difficult and requires specialized imaging techniques that are not available in all hospitals or healthcare settings.

In the United States, the estimated incidence of diagnosed pulmonary embolism is 71 to 117 per 100,000 person-years (5–7), but the true incidence is likely to be much more than this rate because studies show that for every case of diagnosed, non-fatal pulmonary embolism, there are 2.5 cases of fatal pulmonary embolism diagnosed only after death (8). Other studies have estimated that more than one million people in the United States are affected by pulmonary embolism per year, with 100,000 to 200,000 of these events being fatal (5,9).

Over half of all diagnosed cases of pulmonary embolism in the United States occur in patients in hospitals or nursing homes (10). One recent report estimated that more than 12 million patients (31 percent of patients discharged from hospitals in the United States) are at risk of pulmonary embolism (4).

Pulmonary embolism has earned the reputation of a silent killer because less than half of patients who die of pulmonary embolism were diagnosed with the problem prior to death (11).

Risk factors for venous thrombosis and, therefore, pulmonary embolism, include advanced age, prolonged immobility, surgery, trauma, malignancy, pregnancy, estrogen therapy, congestive heart failure, and inherited or acquired defects in blood coagulation factors. These risks are cumulative, putting most hospitalized patients, who often have a combination of these factors, at greater risk of having a pulmonary embolism.

The overall economic burden of pulmonary embolism in the United States is estimated to be over $1.5 billion a year in healthcare costs. Some estimates suggest that pulmonary embolism results in healthcare costs of more than $30,000 per incident (12). Several studies have determined that prevention of pulmonary embolism in hospitalized patients is cost-effective, costing just $3,000 per pulmonary embolism event avoided (13,14).

Pulmonary Embolism

CASE STUDY

A 33-year-old woman was hospitalized for premature labor at 35 weeks of gestation. Labor was successfully stopped, and she was discharged home on strict bed rest. She returned three weeks later in labor. Fetal distress was identified, and an emergency cesarean section resulted in the delivery of a healthy baby. Two days later, the mother reported "crampy" pain in her right leg and was prescribed pain medications. Four days after delivery, she developed sudden shortness of breath and rapid heart rate. A pulmonary embolism was suspected. She was started on the intravenous anticoagulant heparin and underwent a computed tomography (CT) scan with a contrast dye injected into her vein to outline the pulmonary arteries. The resulting images showed a pulmonary embolism, and she was transferred to the intensive care unit. A lower extremity ultrasound found that the source of the embolism was a venous thrombosis in her right thigh. Over the next several days, the patient improved, and she was started on an oral anticoagulation medicine. After a week in the hospital, she returned home, where she recovered fully.

Comment

This patient's risk factors for pulmonary thromboembolism included immobility, the high levels of estrogens associated with pregnancy, and the tissue injury associated with surgery. Her first symptom was subtle and did not immediately suggest venous thrombosis. Once pulmonary embolism was suspected, prompt lifesaving treatment was begun even before the CT scan confirmed the diagnosis. This patient was fortunate not to suffer from complications of the anticoagulant, and the blood clot in her leg was successfully treated. Complications such as bleeding can occur from anticoagulants. Unresolved blood clots can cause chronic pain and swelling in the extremity where the thrombosis occurred. In the lungs, unresolved blood clots can cause increased blood pressure (pulmonary hypertension) and be associated with serious chronic disease. Happily, this patient fully recovered.

What are we learning about this disease?

Pathophysiology, causes, genetics, environment

The delicate balance between coagulation, anticoagulation, and dissolution of clots (thrombolysis) is carefully regulated; any change in cells or clotting factors can upset this balance. Changes may be genetic or acquired. For instance, increased platelets in the blood and abnormal hemoglobin, such as that produced in sickle cell disease, can cause unwanted clotting. Deficiencies in the body's natural anticoagulants, such as protein C and S, can result in thrombus formation, especially if another risk factor is present. Mutations in the clotting factor V increase clotting risk by decreasing the breakdown of this factor. Mutations in factor V are common (present in 5 percent of the population). Abnormalities in thrombolysis, such as deficiencies in antithrombin III, can also promote clot formation.

Anything that reduces blood flow, such as heart failure, narrowing of blood vessels, or immobility, increases the risk for clotting. And almost anything that causes injury, such as cancer, surgery, or trauma, also increases the risk of clot formation.

Annual number of hospitalized patients considered at risk for venous thromboembolism

Discharge diagnosis	n
Heart failure	1,845,319
Respiratory failure	1,490,183
Pneumonia	1,145,469
Cancer	1,039,359
Acute myocardial infarction	577,729
Stroke	507,106
Trauma	419,831
Sepsis	417,875
Arthropathy/spondylopathy	279,261
Paralysis/coma	20,287
Total	7,742,419

The risk of pulmonary embolism depends on the amount of tissue injured and lack of mobility. Brain or nerve tissue injury may be more likely to cause clotting than injuries in other tissue (4).

The greatest risk of pulmonary embolism occurs when a clot has formed in the thighs or pelvis. The blood flow from these areas leads directly to the lungs, where a detached clot can lodge in the pulmonary arteries. Clots in the veins of the calves or arms, however, may also be associated with pulmonary embolism.

How is it prevented, treated, and managed?

Prevention, treatment, staying healthy, prognosis

Preventing venous thrombosis is a major method of preventing pulmonary embolism. People should avoid situations where blood clots might form, such as while staying in a fixed seated position for a long duration in a plane or car. Travelers are encouraged to leave the car or walk around the plane every hour or two and to flex and relax their calf muscles to prevent blood stasis in veins.

In the hospital setting, there is even greater risk because patients often suffer tissue injury and are immobilized in bed. Hospitalized patients are encouraged to get out of bed as soon as possible. Mechanical compression stockings are applied to regularly squeeze the veins in the calf muscles of patients who are not able to walk. Patients are treated with anticoagulants that inhibit one or more of the clotting factors. Although the potential side effects of these measures include bleeding, they have been shown to prevent thrombosis and save lives.

The first step in making a diagnosis is a clinical evaluation that takes into account the risks, symptoms, and signs. Identification of breakdown products of clots in the blood (D-dimers) is a useful biomarker that can further assess the likelihood of a thrombus. An imaging study, usually a chest CT after the injection of a contrast material, outlines the pulmonary arteries and shows a clot if present. Ultrasound of the large veins of the thighs and lower legs may show the presence of clots in these veins. A nuclear medicine lung scan shows areas where no blood flows and is especially good for smaller lung arteries. If the suspicion is very high and the consequences of delayed diagnosis great, anticoagulation may begin even before the tests are done.

Most symptomatic patients with a pulmonary embolism require hospitalization and treatment with anticoagulants. Anticoagulation usually begins with intravenous heparin and is followed by an oral anticoagulant, such as warfarin. Anticoagulation therapy may be prescribed for only a few months or lifelong, depending on the circumstances.

Agents that rapidly break down clots are available. This thrombolytic therapy is usually reserved for severely ill patients because it can cause bleeding. Although infrequent, bleeding into the brain could have dire consequences. In some situations, a filter is placed in the main vein (inferior vena cava) leading from the legs to the lungs to stop any thrombi from traveling to the lungs.

The prognosis depends on the size of the pulmonary embolism. The effect can be so mild as to go unnoticed or it can result in sudden death. If a patient is promptly treated and has no recurrence, it is likely that full function will be restored. Undetected or inadequately treated pulmonary embolism can result in pulmonary hypertension and long-term respiratory disability.

Are we making a difference?

Research past, present, and future

Although the main conditions associated with blood clotting (stasis or slowing of blood flow), hypercoaguability (abnormal clotting factors), and tissue injury were described by the German pathologist Dr. Rudolf Virchow more than 150 years ago, considerable more knowledge on how these affect pulmonary embolism

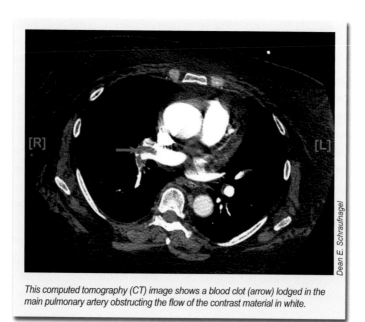

This computed tomography (CT) image shows a blood clot (arrow) lodged in the main pulmonary artery obstructing the flow of the contrast material in white.

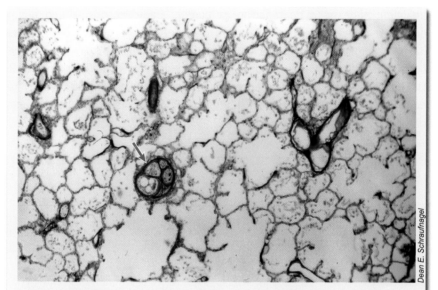

The small pulmonary artery was plugged by a pulmonary embolus. The body organizes and dissolves, or tries to dissolve, the clot to reestablish blood flow (arrow).

has been gained in recent years. Genetic factors associated with blood coagulation problems are being discovered, and more detailed information on the process of blood clotting continues to be learned. It is possible to screen persons for several genetic coagulation abnormalities, although it is uncertain which patients should have these tests performed. Population screening has not been shown to save enough lives or reduce illness sufficiently to justify the expense in most cases.

Research has continued to improve the diagnostic tools, giving better images of the obstructed blood vessels. D-dimer levels appear to be the best of the many diagnostic blood tests studied, although their high sensitivity, which can lead to false positives, is a drawback. D-dimer levels can be elevated in other high-risk situations, such as surgery and certain diseases that cause these products to be found in the blood.

What we need to cure or eliminate pulmonary embolism

Because blood clotting is so important and complex, it is unlikely that pulmonary embolism will ever be eliminated, but progress in diagnosis, prevention, and treatment appears to be reducing its burden. Early recognition and better diagnostic tests may further reduce unexpected death and disability, as well as healthcare costs. Considerable clinical research has attempted to identify the best approach to preventing and treating thrombosis. Several newer anticoagulant drugs are gaining applications because they are either safer, easier to administer, or can be used when side effects from the first-line anticoagulants occur.

References

1. Sandler DA, Martin JF. Autopsy proven pulmonary embolism in hospital patients: are we detecting enough deep vein thrombosis? *J R Soc Med* 1989;82:203–205.
2. Lindblad B, Sternby NH, Bergqvist D. Incidence of venous thromboembolism verified by necropsy over 30 years. *BMJ* 1991;302:709–711.
3. Alikhan R, Peters F, Wilmott R, Cohen AT. Fatal pulmonary embolism in hospitalised patients: a necropsy review. *J Clin Pathol* 2004;57:1254–1257.
4. Anderson FA Jr, Zayaruzny M, Heit JA, Fidan D, Cohen AT. Estimated annual numbers of US acute-care hospital patients at risk for venous thromboembolism. *Am J Hematol* 2007;82:777–782.
5. Anderson FA Jr, Wheeler HB, Goldberg RJ, Hosmer DW, Patwardhan NA, Jovanovic B, Forcier A, Dalen JE. A population-based perspective of the hospital incidence and case-fatality rates of deep vein thrombosis and pulmonary embolism. The Worcester DVT Study. *Arch Intern Med* 1991;151:933–938.
6. Silverstein MD, Heit JA, Mohr DN, Petterson TM, O'Fallon WM, Melton LJ 3rd. Trends in the incidence of deep vein thrombosis and pulmonary embolism: a 25-year population-based study. *Arch Intern Med* 1998;158:585–593.
7. Spencer FA, Emery C, Lessard D, Anderson F, Emani S, Aragam J, Becker RC, Goldberg RJ. The Worcester Venous Thromboembolism study: a population-based study of the clinical epidemiology of venous thromboembolism. *J Gen Intern Med* 2006;21:722–727.
8. Nicolaides AN, Breddin HK, Fareed J, Goldhaber S, Haas S, Hull R, Kalodiki E, Myers K, Samama M, Sasahara A, for the Cardiovascular Disease Educational and Research Trust and the International Union of Angiology. Prevention of venous thromboembolism. International Consensus Statement. Guidelines compiled in accordance with the scientific evidence. *Int Angiol* 2001;20:1–37.
9. Dalen JE, Alpert JS. Natural history of pulmonary embolism. *Prog Cardiovasc Dis* 1975;17:257–270.
10. Heit JA, O'Fallon WM, Petterson TM, Lohse CM, Silverstein MD, Mohr DN, Melton LJ 3rd. Relative impact of risk factors for deep vein thrombosis and pulmonary embolism: a population-based study. *Arch Intern Med* 2002;162:1245–1248.
11. Pineda LA, Hathwar VS, Grant BJ. Clinical suspicion of fatal pulmonary embolism. *Chest* 2001;120:791–795.
12. MacDougall DA, Feliu AL, Boccuzzi SJ, Lin J. Economic burden of deep-vein thrombosis, pulmonary embolism, and post-thrombotic syndrome. *Am J Health Syst Pharm* 2006;63(suppl 6):S5–S15.
13. McGarry LJ, Thompson D, Weinstein MC, Goldhaber SZ. Cost effectiveness of thromboprophylaxis with a low-molecular-weight heparin versus unfractionated heparin in acutely ill medical inpatients. *Am J Manag Care* 2004;10:632–642.
14. Dobesh PP. Economic burden of venous thromboembolism in hospitalized patients. *Pharmacotherapy* 2009;29:943–953.

Web sites of interest

National Institutes of Health
Pulmonary Embolism
www.nlm.nih.gov/medlineplus/pulmonaryembolism.html

Pulmonary Embolus
www.nlm.nih.gov/medlineplus/ency/article/000132.htm

American Heart Association
Circulation Article on Pulmonary Embolism and Deep Vein Thrombosis
www.circ.ahajournals.org/cgi/content/full/106/12/1436

Society for Vascular Surgery
Pulmonary Embolism
www.vascularweb.org/patients/NorthPoint/Pulmonary_Embolism.html

Mayo Clinic
Pulmonary Embolism
www.mayoclinic.com/health/pulmonary-embolism/DS00429

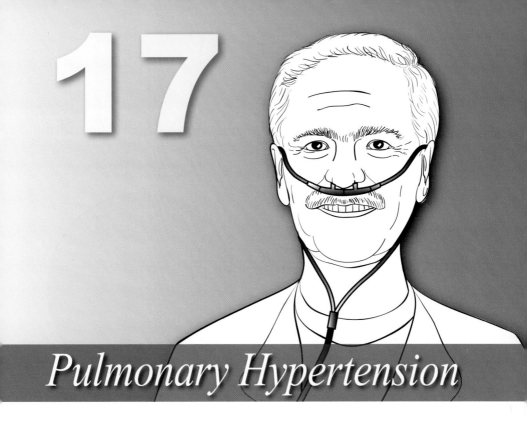

17

Pulmonary Hypertension

Pulmonary hypertension is high blood pressure in the arteries going to the lung. In healthy individuals, the blood pressure in these arteries is much lower than in the rest of the body. In a healthy individual, the blood pressure of the arteries going to the rest of the body is around 120/80 millimeters of mercury (mm Hg) and pulmonary artery blood pressure is about 25/10 mm Hg. If the pulmonary arterial pressure exceeds about 40/20 mm Hg or the average pressure exceeds 25 mm Hg, then pulmonary hypertension is present. If pulmonary hypertension persists or becomes very high, the right ventricle of the heart, which supplies blood to the pulmonary arteries, is unable to pump effectively, and the person experiences symptoms that include shortness of breath, loss of energy, and edema, which is a sign of *right* heart failure. Many diseases and conditions increase the pulmonary artery pressure.

Whom does it affect?

Epidemiology, prevalence, economic burden, vulnerable populations

The exact prevalence of all types of pulmonary hypertension in the United States and the world is not known. The number of patients in the United States is certainly in the hundreds of thousands, with many more who are undiagnosed. About 200,000 hospitalizations occur annually in the United States with

Causes of pulmonary arterial hypertension

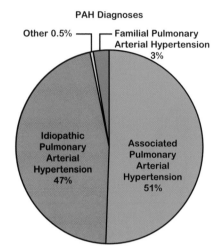

PAH Diagnoses

Other 0.5% ── ┌── Familial Pulmonary
                  Arterial Hypertension
                  3%

Idiopathic Pulmonary Arterial Hypertension 47%

Associated Pulmonary Arterial Hypertension 51%

Diseases associated with pulmonary arterial hypertension

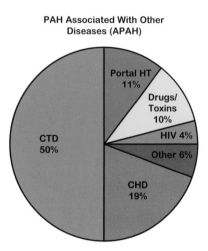

PAH Associated With Other Diseases (APAH)

Portal HT 11%

Drugs/ Toxins 10%

HIV 4%

Other 6%

CTD 50%

CHD 19%

The pie chart on the left shows the causes of pulmonary arterial hypertension. The pie chart on the right breaks down the diseases associated with it. (Chronic thromboembolic pulmonary hypertension was not part of this registry.) Portal HT is pulmonary hypertension associated with liver disease. CTD is connective tissue disease; CHD is congenital heart disease. Reprinted from the *Journal of the American College of Cardiology,* Vol. 53. Issue 17, "ACCF/AHA 2009 Expert Consensus Document on Pulmonary Hypertension: A Report of the American College of Cardiology Foundation Task Force on Expert Consensus Documents and the American Heart Association," with permission from Elsevier.

pulmonary hypertension as a primary or secondary diagnosis (1). About 15,000 deaths per year are ascribed to pulmonary hypertension, although this is certainly a low estimate (1). Most medical references to heart failure are for *left* heart failure, which in the United States has a prevalence of about 4.9 million and an annual incidence of 378 per 100,000 (2,3). Pulmonary hypertension, which causes right heart failure, affects all races and socioeconomic levels.

The most common cause of pulmonary hypertension in the developing world is schistosomiasis, a parasitic infection in which the parasite's eggs can lodge in and obstruct the pulmonary arteries. Another risk factor for pulmonary hypertension is high altitude. More than 140 million persons worldwide and up to 1 million in the United States live 10,000 feet or more above sea level (4). In African Americans, sickle cell anemia is an important cause of pulmonary hypertension.

A specific type of pulmonary hypertension in which the disease process occurs in the pulmonary arteries themselves is called *pulmonary arterial hypertension*

Pulmonary Hypertension

CASE STUDY

A 28-year-old woman had felt well and worked full time in landscape design until she noticed she was becoming short of breath when she exerted herself. She noted a dry cough and had leg swelling. She had a total loss of energy, which was devastating because she was so active. She was diagnosed with pulmonary arterial hypertension (PAH) due to congenital heart disease, and because of her advanced right heart failure, she was started on intravenous epoprostenol therapy. The severity of her disease came as a surprise to her and her family, and she struggled to cope with the new medications and management regimen, especially sodium restriction. Being told that she would not be able to bear children brought great sadness to her, but she felt fortunate to have nieces and nephews to spend time with. Like many people, she researched her disease and prognosis on the Internet, which was both empowering but also, frankly, terrifying. She nonetheless remained positive about her future.

Comment

This case is a common presentation of pulmonary hypertension: a previously healthy young woman develops a life-threatening disease with no outward manifestation. Because these patients look normal at rest, friends, family, and coworkers have a difficult time accepting that they are sick. The advent of newer drugs has doubled survival for PAH, and many patients are now living well beyond a decade with reasonable function and satisfaction.

(PAH). This condition generally affects young and otherwise healthy individuals and strikes women twice as frequently as men. The average age of diagnosis is 36 years, and three-year survival after diagnosis is only about 50 percent. Each year, between 10 and 15 people per million population are diagnosed with the disease. With improved treatments and survival, the number of U.S. patients living with the disease has increased to between 10,000 and 20,000 (5).

Because so many disorders can result in severe pulmonary hypertension and treatments may vary dramatically, it is important for a thorough evaluation to occur when pulmonary hypertension is detected or suspected. For instance, pulmonary hypertension related to blood clots in the pulmonary arteries (pulmonary embolism and thromboembolic pulmonary hypertension) requires anticoagulation and, in some cases, surgical removal of the clots. Because about 250,000 cases of pulmonary embolism occur each year in the United States, thousands of patients are annually at risk of residual pulmonary hypertension from this disorder (6). The actual number is not easily determined because most cases of pulmonary embolism go undiagnosed.

What are we learning about pulmonary hypertension?

Pathophysiology, causes: genetic, environment, microbes

The last 20 years have witnessed an explosion of clinical and research advances in pulmonary arterial hypertension (PAH) that have resulted from better understanding of the mechanisms of the disease. A genetic cause of PAH was found by two groups in 2000, and it has led to research and increased understanding of the condition. Mutations in an oddly named receptor, bone morphogenetic protein receptor type 2 (BMPR2), are the cause of heritable PAH in over

Surviving pulmonary arterial hypertension

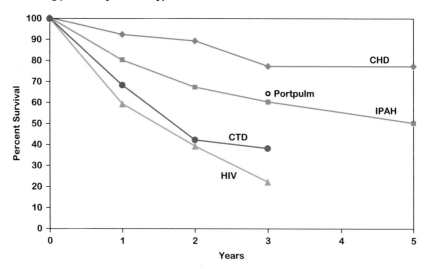

Survival in PAH after diagnosis in patients with existing CHD (congenital heart disease), Portpulm (portapulmonary disease), IPAH (idiopathic pulmonary hypertension), CTD (connective tissue disease), and HIV in the mid-2000s. Adapted from (2).

Pulmonary Hypertension

Pulmonary hypertension by mechanism of disease

Due to left heart failure (increased back pressure in the pulmonary vessels)

- Left ventricular pump failure (heart attack, cardiomyopathy)
- Left ventricular stiffness (hypertension, diabetes, metabolic syndrome)
- Valve disease (mitral or aortic stenosis or regurgitation)

Diseases affecting the whole lung (lung diseases obliterate blood vessels)

- Chronic bronchitis and emphysema (combination of loss of lung plus hypoxia)
- Interstitial lung diseases (destructive diseases that obliterate vessels, such as pulmonary fibrosis, sarcoidosis, and many others)

Hypoxia related (decreased oxygen constricts pulmonary blood vessels)

- High-altitude dwelling
- Sleep apnea and other hypoventilation syndromes
- Hypoxia of chronic bronchitis and emphysema (chronic obstructive pulmonary disease, or COPD)

Pulmonary arterial hypertension (changes in the structure and function of the pulmonary arteries)

- Idiopathic (formerly primary pulmonary hypertension)
- Heritable (formerly familial, due to BMPR2 or Alk-1 mutations)
- Drug- and toxin-induced (stimulants)
- Connective tissue diseases (especially scleroderma)
- HIV infection (rare occurrence <1%)
- Portal hypertension (cirrhosis and other advanced liver diseases)
- Congenital heart disease that allows blood to shunt around the lungs
- Pulmonary veno-occlusive disease and pulmonary capillary hemangiomatosis (rare)

Primarily obstructing diseases of the pulmonary vessels

- Pulmonary thromboembolism
- Schistosomiasis
- Sickle cell anemia
- Tumor emboli
- Fibrosing mediastinitis (obstruction by fibrosis related to histoplasmosis)

85 percent of afflicted families. BMPR2 mutations are found in about 10 to 20 percent of people with PAH who have no other family members with the disease. It is now known that multiple biological pathways lead to PAH, and, therefore, different drug treatments may ultimately benefit specific types of patients.

In addition, PAH has been associated with connective tissue diseases (especially scleroderma), liver disease (portapulmonary hypertension), human immunodeficiency virus (HIV) infection, congenital heart disease, and stimulant drug ingestion. However, the most common type of PAH is idiopathic—with no known cause.

Little is known about the effect of the environment or microbes on pulmonary hypertension, although molecular mediators of inflammation interact with many molecules that affect changes in pulmonary blood vessels. Stimulants such as amphetamines, the erstwhile diet pill fenfluramine/phentermine (Fenphen), methamphetamine, and cocaine can cause or exacerbate pulmonary hypertension.

How is it prevented, treated, and managed?

Prevention, treatment, staying healthy, prognosis

There is no way to prevent pulmonary hypertension, although drugs and toxins that cause or worsen the disease should be avoided.

Because it is best detected and measured by echocardiography or right heart catheterization—tests that most patients do not undergo—pulmonary hypertension is generally not diagnosed until the disease is advanced and the right heart begins to fail. By then, the disease is usually incurable.

In some patients with pulmonary arterial hypertension (PAH), vasodilator drugs, such as calcium channel blockers, reduce pulmonary hypertension and improve quality of life. Unfortunately, only a minority of patients—less than 10 percent—benefit from this therapy. Also, PAH usually involves the accumulation of fibrous tissue in the pulmonary arteries, a problem not amenable to vasodilation.

Understanding of the physiology of the blood vessels in the lungs has led to the development and testing of several new classes of drugs. These drugs have vasodilator potential but also other beneficial characteristics, including platelet inhibition, anti-smooth muscle proliferation, and improved cardiac function. The

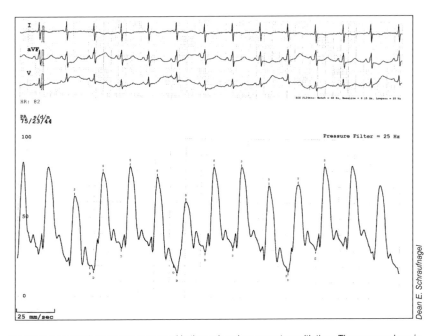

This tracing shows the pressure measured in the main pulmonary artery with time. The pressure here is about 82/18 mm Hg. Normal pressure is about 25/10 mm Hg.

overall survival of patients with idiopathic PAH has doubled with these drugs, and quality of life has markedly improved.

In addition to the calcium channel blockers, three other classes of vasoactive drugs are used to treat pulmonary hypertension: endothelin receptor antagonists, phosphodiesterase-5 inhibitors, and prostaglandins (of which prostacyclin is the most important). Endothelin receptor antagonists block the endothelin effects of vasoconstriction and smooth muscle growth. Phosphodiesterase-5 inhibitors address the relative lack of nitric oxide in patients with PAH. Nitric oxide is a potent relaxer of the blood vessels. There are minimal side effects with this class and, similar to the endothelin receptor antagonists, these drugs are moderately effective in treating pulmonary hypertension. The first fully effective treatment for PAH was the prostacyclin derivative epoprostenol, which was approved in 1995. It has been shown to improve survival in this disease, but it has many side effects, like flushing, jaw pain, and nausea.

Although each of these classes of drugs is a major advance in the therapy of PAH, a proportion of patients will continue to worsen despite treatment with the best drugs. These patients may be candidates for lung transplantation or, very rarely, for a procedure called *atrial septostomy,* which creates a connection from the right side of the heart to the left side to allow blood to bypass the lungs.

Staying healthy with most forms of pulmonary hypertension can often be challenging. Patients must work with their healthcare team. Drug regimens often require frequent dosing and have many side effects. In addition, patients with heart failure are usually asked to follow a low-salt diet and to limit the amount of liquids they drink daily. Because patients with pulmonary hypertension cannot tolerate the stress of pregnancy, women of childbearing age are generally told not to get pregnant and are encouraged to be sterilized. Patients whose pulmonary artery pressure significantly improves with a vasodilator have a much better prognosis.

Are we making a difference?

Research past, present, and future

The accurate diagnosis and effective management of pulmonary hypertension is a medical triumph made possible by the development of right heart catheterization

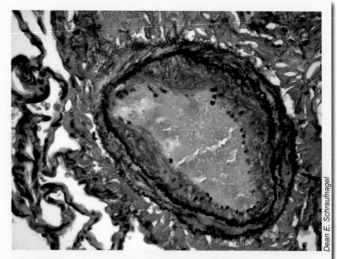

This microscopic view of a small pulmonary artery shows that its inner lining (endothelium) extends into the center of the vessel. This is a common early change in pulmonary arterial hypertension.

in the 1940s. In 1951, the entity "primary pulmonary hypertension" was accurately described. A major advance was the development of Doppler echocardiography, which allowed noninvasive imaging of the right ventricle and estimation of pulmonary artery pressure. The discovery that calcium channel blockers were occasionally extremely effective in idiopathic pulmonary arterial hypertension (PAH) and that intravenous prostacyclin not only dramatically improved quality of life but also doubled survival stimulated research into the development of other agents.

The genetic revolution, funded by the National Institutes of Health and other agencies, led to the discovery of the genes responsible for heritable pulmonary hypertension and is leading to the identification of other genes that may permit or modify disease. These discoveries have resulted in more awareness of the intricate and complicated interactions of various cells and their metabolic pathways. The biological revolution in intracellular signaling and cell-to-cell communication has led to insights into the mechanisms of disease. New drugs are being developed and tested for beneficial effects. Because of the hope engendered by these advances, patient- and family-centered associations, such as the Pulmonary Hypertension Association, have become forces for education, research, and service to people affected by pulmonary hypertension and professionals dedicated to defeating the disease.

What we need to cure or eliminate pulmonary hypertension

Better tests are needed to make an early diagnosis. The tests should be convenient for screening and could identify persons at risk or give a measure of how severe the disease is. They could be in the form of genetic markers, which could identify risk, or of blood hormones or mediators, such as brain natriuretic peptide, that might rise with worsening disease. What is currently available, however, does not adequately assess either risk or severity.

Further research will be needed to produce safer and more effective drugs that one day may be used in presymptomatic patients at high risk for pulmonary hypertension, such as those with scleroderma or those who have family members with pulmonary hypertension. Although there is much more to be done, the future has never been brighter.

References

1. Hyduk A, Croft JB, Ayala C, Zheng K, Zheng ZJ, Mensah GA. Pulmonary hypertension surveillance—United States, 1980–2002. *MMWR Surveill Summ* 2005;54:1–28.
2. Hunt SA, Baker DW, Chin MH, Cinquegrani MP, Feldman AM, Francis GS, Ganiats TG, Goldstein S, Gregoratos G, Jessup ML, et al; for the American College of Cardiology/ American Heart Association. ACC/AHA guidelines for the evaluation and management of chronic heart failure in the adult: executive summary. A report of the American College of Cardiology/American Heart Association Task Force on Practice Guidelines (Committee to revise the 1995 Guidelines for the Evaluation and Management of Heart Failure). *J Am Coll Cardiol* 2001;38:2101–2113.
3. Roger VL, Weston SA, Redfield MM, Hellermann-Homan JP, Killian J, Yawn BP, Jacobsen SJ. Trends in heart failure incidence and survival in a community-based population. *JAMA* 2004;292:344–350.
4. Penaloza D, Arias-Stella J. The heart and pulmonary circulation at high altitudes: healthy highlanders and chronic mountain sickness. *Circulation* 2007;115:1132–1146.
5. Badesch DB, Raskob GE, Elliott CG, Krichman AM, Farber HW, Frost AE, Barst RJ, Benza RL, Liou TG, Turner M, et al. Pulmonary arterial hypertension: baseline characteristics from the REVEAL Registry. *Chest* 2010;137:376–387.
6. Silverstein MD, Heit JA, Mohr DN, Petterson TM, O'Fallon WM, Melton LJ 3rd. Trends in the incidence of deep vein thrombosis and pulmonary embolism: a 25-year population-based study. *Arch Intern Med* 1998;158:585–593.

Web sites of interest

National Institutes of Health Medline Plus
Pulmonary Hypertension
www.nlm.nih.gov/medlineplus/pulmonaryhypertension.html

American Heart Association
Pulmonary Hypertension
www.americanheart.org/presenter.jhtml?identifier=11076

Pulmonary Hypertension Association
www.phassociation.org

18

Rare Lung Diseases

A rare disease is defined by the U.S. National Institutes of Health Office of Rare Diseases as one that affects fewer than 200,000 people in the United States. However, there are between 5,000 and 8,000 distinct rare disorders that, together, affect more than 20 million people in the United States. A conservative estimate of primary or secondary lung involvement in 5 to 10 percent of rare diseases suggests that there are at least 1 to 2 million American patients suffering from rare lung diseases (1,2).

Whom does it affect?

Epidemiology, prevalence, economic burden, vulnerable populations

As a group, uncommon lung diseases affect at least 1 in every 200 persons. Examples of rare lung diseases include sarcoidosis (see Chapter 21), an inflammatory disorder often affecting the lungs and other organs; alpha-1 antitrypsin deficiency, a genetic disorder that leads to emphysema; lymphangioleiomyomatosis (LAM), a cystic lung disease; many congenital lung disorders; a group of lung diseases affecting the blood vessels (vasculitis); rare tumors that involve the lung; rare infectious diseases such as the plague; and other disorders of

The most "common" rare lung diseases

A	More than 1 per 100,000	
B	1–10 per million	
C	Dozens to hundreds of case reports	
D	Isolated case reports	

Infectious diseases

Fibrosing mediastinitis		C

Phakomatoses

Birt-Hogg-Dube		B
Lymphangioleiomyomatosis		B
Neurofibromatosis type I (with lung involvement)		C

Inherited forms of emphysema

Alpha-1 antitrypsin deficiency		A
Elastin mutations		D
Salla disease		D

Pulmonary vascular diseases

Familial pulmonary arterial hypertension		A
Pulmonary alveolar proteinosis		B
Pulmonary capillary hemangiomatosis		C
Pulmonary veno-occlusive disease		C
Hereditary hemorrhagic telangiectasia (with lung involvement)		A

Channelopathies

Pulmonary alveolar microlithiasis		C
Cystic fibrosis		A

Ciliary disorders

Kartagener syndrome		B
Primary ciliary dyskinesia		B

(continued on next page)

Rare Lung Diseases

Disorders of respiratory drive

Central alveolar hypoventilation	C
Narcolepsy	A

Connective tissue matrix disorders

Marfan syndrome (with lung involvement)	C
Ehler–Danlos syndrome (with lung involvement)	C

Genetic surfactant disorders

ABCA3	C
SP-A-related lung disease	D
SP-B-related lung disease	C
SP-C-related lung disease	C

Trafficking and lysosomal storage disorders

Hermansky–Pudlak syndrome	B
Gaucher disease (with lung involvement)	C
Neiman Pick C (with lung involvement)	C

Vasculitis

Wegener's granulomatosis	A
Goodpasture syndrome	B
Microscopic polyangiitis (with lung involvement)	B
Polyarteritis nodosa (with lung involvement)	B
Churg–Strauss syndrome	A

Congenital

Cystic adenomatoid malformation	C
Pulmonary sequestration	C
Neuroendocrine cell hyperplasia	B

Neuromuscular disease

Amyotrophic lateral sclerosis	A

(continued on next page)

Myasthenia gravis	A
Dermatomyositis, polymyositis	A
Other	
Sarcoidosis	A
Langerhans cell histiocytosis	B
Idiopathic pulmonary hemosiderosis	C
Sickle cell anemia (with lung involvement)	A
Lymphangiomatosis	C

Data from the Office of Rare Diseases and Orphanet (1,2).

which the cause and cellular defect may be known or unknown. Diseases of unknown etiology are termed *idiopathic*.

The prevalence of rare lung disorders varies widely by disease type. The lungs may also be involved as a rare manifestation of another more common disorder, such as Marfan syndrome. Some lung diseases are so rare that they only have been described in case reports. The most "common" rare lung diseases, as defined by the Office of Rare Diseases and Orphanet, occur in up to 70 patients per 100,000 (1,2).

Estimating the economic burden of rare lung disease is difficult. As a group comprising 1 to 2 million affected persons, and with a conservative estimate of average yearly healthcare expenditures of $5,000 per patient, the annual total cost is in the billions of dollars. The rarer the disorder, the more tests and healthcare

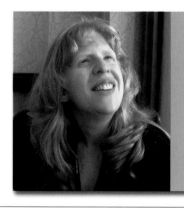

Ashley Appell, who is 23 years old, has Hermansky–Pudlak syndrome, a rare genetic disease associated with albinism, a bleeding disorder caused by abnormal platelets, and interstitial lung disease.

Rare Lung Diseases

visits are likely required to arrive at the correct diagnosis. These delays result in greater expenses, unnecessary tests, and missed opportunities for early intervention. For example, the average interval from onset of symptoms to the diagnosis of LAM, which affects smooth muscle tissue in the lungs and airways, is three to five years (3). Most patients suffer two episodes of pneumothorax (collapsed lung) before the diagnosis is made. Misdiagnosis as primary spontaneous pneumothorax, asthma, or chronic obstructive lung disease (COPD) leads to inappropriate care and increased risk (for instance, uninformed decisions regarding pregnancy and air travel). Rare diseases are in many cases serious, chronic, and debilitating, and, once properly diagnosed, often require expensive, long-term treatments.

Rare lung diseases generally affect individuals from birth through about age 60, and are uncommon in the elderly. Some diseases are more prevalent in certain racial and ethnic populations, such as sarcoidosis in African Americans, for unknown reasons. For rare genetic lung diseases, there may be great regional variation, such as cystic fibrosis (1 in 350,000 in Japan vs. 1 in 10,000 in the United States), Hermansky–Pudlak syndrome, a disease associated with albinism, bleeding, and lung scarring (1 in 1,800 in Puerto Rico vs. only isolated case reports and small clusters in the rest of the world), and pulmonary alveolar microlithiasis, a disease associated with sand-like particles in the lung, which occurs predominantly in Japan and Turkey (4).

What we are learning about rare lung diseases?

Pathophysiology, causes: genetic, environment, microbes

The causes and pathophysiology of these diseases are varied and complex. Many have a genetic basis, and most diseases have genetic influence. The environment and micro organisms may play a role, especially in those diseases in which the patient's immune defense has been compromised. Further description of individual diseases and how they have helped researchers learn about other diseases is discussed in the last section of this chapter.

How are they prevented, treated, and managed?

Prevention, treatment, staying healthy, prognosis

Given the number and diversity of rare diseases of the lungs and other organs, it is not feasible for primary care physicians to become informed about all of

CASE STUDY

A 38-year-old woman with a history of excessive menstrual bleeding, vision impairment easy bruising, and involuntary movement of the eyes (nystagmus) complained of an upper respiratory infection and sought medical attention when her cough would not go away. She was treated with antibiotics, but her symptoms persisted. A chest radiograph was abnormal, and a computed tomography (CT) scan of the chest showed fibrosis, or lung scarring. Idiopathic pulmonary fibrosis was diagnosed with a surgical lung biopsy. Post-procedure bleeding complicated her recovery. Her ability to exercise progressively declined, and she became oxygen dependent. A family member, concerned about her rapid deterioration, searched for answers on the Internet. The history of bruising, heavy menstrual cycles, and fair skin suggested a possible diagnosis of Hermansky–Pudlak syndrome, as did the pulmonary fibrosis itself. At the request of her family, a blood test was ordered to examine her platelets under an electron microscope. A lack of platelet-dense bodies was confirmed, and the diagnosis of Hermansky–Pudlak syndrome was made (5). Clinical deterioration continued, and within a year, the patient received a lung transplant.

Comment

Rare diseases by their nature are difficult to diagnose. Most patients are labeled with a common disease and treated, often inappropriately, for prolonged periods before the correct diagnosis is made. Had the diagnosis in the patient above been made earlier, the lung biopsy, risky because of the patient's propensity to bleed, could have been averted. This patient's correct diagnosis allowed her family members to be screened for the syndrome and prevented further diagnostic confusion.

The healthcare burden of rare disease is often greater than that of more common diseases. Doctors may not have seen the disease before. Patients may become frustrated being undiagnosed or discouraged because they do not "fit" the erroneous diagnosis they have been given. Tests may be unusual and difficult to obtain, and insurers may not cover those tests. Researchers may not prioritize rare diseases. Employers may be unfamiliar with the disease and may not adequately respect the disability of the patient. Patients with rare diseases often drive the diagnostic process forward, and patient advocacy organizations play an essential role in the rare lung disease community.

them, but it is important that primary care training include guidance on the recognition and referral of lung disorders that fall outside the spectrum of common disorders. It is equally important that pulmonary specialty training incorporate education about the rarest lung disorders. Once the diagnosis is made, referral to centers with focused expertise in that particular rare lung disease is often advisable. Many of the rare lung diseases caused by a single, mutated gene, such as alpha-1 antitrypsin deficiency, surfactant protein (SP) disorders, and cystic fibrosis, lend themselves to family screening, including genetic analysis. Diseases identified at an early stage in this way are more apt to be properly treated, and are more likely reversible than diseases not diagnosed until later stages.

The basic principles of lung health also apply to rare lung disorders, including not smoking, avoidance of noxious occupational environmental exposures, and regular exercise. Patients should have periodic follow-up physician visits.

Treatment of rare lung diseases often involves the use of unconventional therapies and orphan drugs, such as subcutaneous injections of granulocyte macrophage colony–stimulating factor (GM-CSF) for pulmonary alveolar proteinosis (6), glucocerebrosidase therapy for Gaucher disease, and alpha-1 antitrypsin replacement for hereditary emphysema. (An orphan drug is one that treats rare, or "orphan" diseases and would not ordinarily be profitable for pharmaceutical companies to develop. Support to develop these drugs was advanced by the Orphan Drug Act of 1983.) In other cases, simply removing the trigger may be sufficient, such as smoking cessation in patients with Langerhans cell histiocytosis.

The prognosis for patients with rare lung diseases is as variable as the diseases themselves. A baby born with surfactant protein B deficiency will die in infancy, while children born today with cystic fibrosis have a good chance of celebrating their 35th birthday.

Are we making a difference?

Research past, present, and future

Some of the most exciting discoveries in pulmonary medicine have come from studying rare diseases. Insights gained from uncommon lung diseases often shed light on more common lung diseases, as illustrated by the examples below (7).

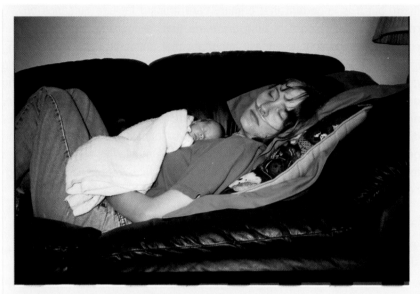

Young women are the victims of LAM. This photograph of a mother and her baby poignantly illustrates that fact that young women can be the victim of rare lung diseases.

Insights into pulmonary fibrosis

Two rare disease—surfactant protein C deficiency and Hermansky–Pudlak syndrome—are helping researchers understand pulmonary fibrosis.

Mutations in surfactant protein C, a protein that is produced only in one cell type in the lung's alveoli, result in respiratory failure in infants and a predisposition to pulmonary fibrosis in adulthood (8). Because of this rare disease, it is known that the alveolar lining cells play a primary role in the cause and progression of pulmonary fibrosis, most likely through protein misfolding. (After proteins are produced, they must be transported to the place where they have their effect and must be properly folded or shaped to make the journey and perform their function.)

Hermansky–Pudlak syndrome is caused by mutations in genes that control the movement of molecules between stations within the cell (5). Tracking the development of lung scarring in these patients and understanding the cause of lung scarring from the vantage point of the primary molecular defect promises to shed light on how more common forms of lung fibrosis occur.

Rare Lung Diseases

Insights into metastatic cancer

Lymphangioleiomyomatosis (LAM) is a cystic lung disease of women that is associated with mutations in genes that control cell energy utilization, growth and movement (3). The lungs become invaded by destructive, mutant cells that originate from an unknown, remote source. In essence, LAM is a very slowly moving metastatic neoplasm caused by a single genetic mutation; as such, the study of LAM may yield insights into the cellular and molecular basis of all cancers.

Insights into pulmonary defense against infections

Pulmonary alveolar proteinosis (PAP) is caused by an autoantibody that neutralizes the function of a molecule called *granulocyte macrophage colony–stimulating factor* (GM-CSF) (6). GM-CSF is important for the antimicrobial function of white blood cells. The absence of GM-CSF function results in the failure of cells in the lung to clear pulmonary surfactant, the oily material that lines the airspaces and keeps them open during respiration. GM-CSF is also important for the antimicrobial function of white blood cells. As a result, in the absence of GM-CSF action surfactant lipids and proteins accumulate in the airspace, and infections can occur both in the lung and other parts of the body. Understanding of the mechanisms of PAP has shown the central role that GM-CSF plays in the regulation of surfactant and other components of the complex biological systems in lung host defense. GM-CSF is being developed as an immunity-enhancing treatment for several diseases.

Insights into pulmonary homeostasis

Pulmonary surfactant contains special chemicals called *phospholipids*, which must be synthesized and metabolized in a balanced, tightly regulated fashion. The cause behind the accumulation of tiny, sand-like calcium phosphate granules in the lungs of patients with a rare condition known as *pulmonary alveolar microlithiasis* was a complete mystery (4). That is, until scientists in Japan discovered that the gene involved was the sole alveolar phosphate transporter (a transporter is a molecule or set of molecules that spans a cell membrane and moves ions, such as potassium or calcium, across the membrane against a gradient). We now know that phosphate byproducts of phospholipid metabolism are cleared by a transporter on alveolar type II cells (called *SLC34A2*). A rare disease revealed a biological truth that otherwise would have taken decades to learn.

What we need to cure and eliminate rare lung diseases

Realizing the value of this type of research, the National Institutes of Health (NIH) has fostered basic research on rare diseases. In 2003, the NIH established the Rare Lung Disease Consortium to conduct cooperative trials and inform the public about the less common lung disorders. Engaging pharmaceutical firms in the development of orphan drugs for rare diseases often facilitates the availability of drugs for other disorders.

Patient advocacy organizations are valuable allies in the fight against rare lung disease, by educating, supporting, and organizing patients and families in a manner that facilitates research. The development of central databases, registries, and research networks are useful adjuncts. With such rare disorders, international cooperation is critical for accumulating sufficient numbers of patients for research.

Additional referral centers for patients with rare lung diseases are needed to provide multidisciplinary, expert care. Development of educational materials enhances the recognition and visibility of rare lung diseases with patients, health professionals, and the general public. Training professionals to recognize, refer, diagnose, and treat rare lung diseases is also needed.

References

1. Orphanet Web site. About rare diseases. Available at: http://www.orpha.net/consor/cgi-bin/ Education_AboutRareDiseases.php?Ing=EN. Accessed July 2009.
2. National Institutes of Health Office of Rare Diseases Research Web site. Home page. Available at: http://rarediseases.info.nih.gov?AboutUsAspx. Accessed July 2009. .
3. McCormack FX. Lymphangioleiomyomatosis: a clinical update. *Chest* 2008;133:507–516.
4. Huqun SI, Miyazawa H, Ishii K, Uchiyama B, Ishida T, Tanaka S, Tazawa R, Fukuyama S, Tanaka T, Nagai Y, et al. Mutations in the *SLC34A2* gene are associated with pulmonary alveolar microlithiasis. *Am J Respir Crit Care Med* 2007;175:263–268.
5. Huizing M, Anikster Y, Gahl WA. Hermansky–Pudlak syndrome and related disorders of organelle formation. *Traffic* 2000;1:823–835.
6. Trapnell BC, Whitsett JA, Nakata K. Pulmonary alveolar proteinosis. *N Engl J Med* 2003;349:2527–2539.
7. McCormack FX, Panos RJ, Trapnell BC, eds. *Molecular Basis of Pulmonary Disease: Insights from Rare Lung Disorders*. New York, NY: Humana Press; Springer Science and Business Media, LLC 2010.
8. Tager AM, Sharma A, Mark EJ. Case records of the Massachusetts General Hospital. Case 32-2009. A 27-year-old man with progressive dyspnea. *N Engl J Med* 2009;361: 1585–1593.

Web sites of interest

National Institutes of Health Rare Diseases Clinical Research Network
www.rarediseasesnetwork.org
Orphanet
About Rare Diseases
www.orpha.net/consor/cgi-bin/Education_AboutRareDiseases.php?Ing=EN

LAM Foundation
www.thelamfoundation.org

Hermansky-Pudlak Syndrome Network
www.hermansky-pudlak.org

Tuberous Sclerosis Alliance
www.tsalliance.org

19

Respiratory Distress Syndrome of the Newborn

Respiratory distress syndrome (RDS) of the newborn, also known as *hyaline membrane disease*, is a breathing disorder of premature babies. In healthy infants, the alveoli—the small, air-exchanging sacs of the lungs—are coated by surfactant, which is a soap-like material produced in the lungs as the fetus matures in preparation for birth. If premature newborns have not yet produced enough surfactant, they are unable to open their lungs fully to breathe.

Whom does it affect?

Epidemiology, prevalence, economic burden, and vulnerable populations

Respiratory distress syndrome (RDS) affects about 1 percent of newborn infants and is the leading cause of death in babies who are born prematurely (1). About 12 percent of babies born in the United States are preterm, which is higher than in other developed countries (2). About 10 percent of premature babies in the United States develop RDS each year (3). The risk of RDS rises with increasing prematurity. Babies born before 29 weeks of gestation have a 60 percent chance of developing RDS (4), but babies born at full term rarely develop this condition. Maternal risk factors for preterm birth include previous preterm birth, periodontal disease, low maternal body mass, poor prenatal care, poverty, being uninsured, and being a member of a minority group (5).

Respiratory distress syndrome in the United States by birth weight

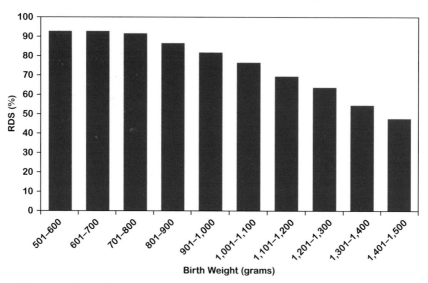

Incidence of respiratory distress syndrome (RDS) in the United States relative to birth weight, which shows it is a disease of premature infants. Horbar JD, Carpenter JH, Kenny M, eds. Vermont Oxford Network 2002 Very Low Birth Weight Database Summary. Burlington, VT: Vermont Oxford Network; 2003.

Among premature babies, the risk of developing RDS increases with Caucasian race, male sex, an older sibling with RDS, cesarean delivery, perinatal asphyxia, and maternal diabetes.

In 2003, the total number of live births in the United States for all races was 4,089,950; about 0.6 percent of newborns had RDS (about 24,000 or 6 per 1,000 live births) (6). In 2005, there were 4,138,000 live births in the United States, and a slightly larger number of babies were affected with RDS because the rate of premature births had increased from 11.6 percent to 12.7 percent, mainly due to a rise in late preterm births (34 to 36 weeks of gestation) (7).

Even though the number of RDS cases in the United States is growing, the infant mortality rate from RDS has dramatically declined from about 25,000 deaths per year in the 1960s to 860 deaths in 2005 (7) because of surfactant replacement therapy. Infant deaths from RDS were 2.6 times greater in African American babies than in Caucasian babies, although Caucasian babies are at a higher risk to develop the condition.

In 2001, hospital charges for a premature baby were estimated to be $75,000 (8). With approximately 18,000 hospitalizations each year due to

Respiratory Distress Syndrome

CASE STUDY

In August 1963, First Lady Jacqueline Bouvier Kennedy was hospitalized in her 34th week of pregnancy at the Otis Air Force Base Hospital. Her fetus was in distress, but labor did not progress. On August 7, she underwent a cesarean section to deliver Patrick Bouvier Kennedy, who weighed 4 pounds, 10.5 ounces (2,112 grams). After delivery, the baby developed difficulty breathing, which did not improve despite oxygen therapy. The baby was then rushed to Children's Hospital Boston, a leading center in respiratory distress syndrome (RDS). Unfortunately, despite the best medical efforts, the baby died two days later. The death of the newborn baby devastated the First Family. In the weeks that followed the tragedy, the president and his mother-in-law, Janet Auchincloss, feared that Jacqueline would have a nervous breakdown, although it was reported that this adversity ultimately brought the president and his wife closer together.

Comment

Although RDS affects the infant, in many ways, it takes a greater toll on the families. The newborn may be in a neonatal intensive care unit for a prolonged period, and the outcome is likely to be death or lifelong disability. The emotional, family, and economic stress can be ruinous. The story of the Kennedy child gripped the nation and alerted the world to the dire consequences of infant RDS. Patrick Kennedy's obituary in the New York Times *stated that the only treatment "for a victim of hyaline membrane disease is to monitor the infant's blood chemistry and to try to keep it near normal levels. Thus, the battle for the Kennedy baby was lost only because medical science has not yet advanced far enough to accomplish as quickly as necessary what the body can do by itself in its own time."*

RDS, the total cost of treating these babies in the hospital is approximately $2.3 billion.

What we are learning about the disease

Pathophysiology, causes: genetic, environment, microbes

Through the ages, infant death has been attributed to an inability of the newborn to adapt to life outside the uterus. In the early 20th century, "hyaline membranes" were found during autopsy in the lungs of infants who died shortly after birth, but never in stillborns. In the 1920s, Dr. Kurt von Neergaard, a Swiss physiologist, postulated the existence of a substance in the lungs that reduces surface tension, allowing the lungs to open. In the 1950s, Dr. John Clements, a U.S. pulmonary physiologist, showed that this substance was surfactant. Finally, in 1959, Drs. Mary Ellen Avery and Jere Mead, both working at Harvard at the time, demonstrated that surfactant was lacking in the lungs of premature babies, which was the base cause of the respiratory failure seen in some of these infants (9).

Further study on infant respiratory distress syndrome (RDS) found that the deficiency of surfactant was a consequence of either insufficient production by the immature lungs or a genetic mutation in one of the surfactant proteins, SP-B. The rarer genetic form of the disease is not associated with premature birth and occurs in full-term babies (10).

Surfactant is necessary for the tiny lung alveoli to overcome surface tension and remain open. Without adequate surfactant, the pressure exerted trying to open these alveoli by either the baby's desperate breathing or by a mechanical ventilator ruptures the alveoli, producing an emphysema-like picture, or pneumothorax, if the air escapes outside the lung and is trapped in the chest wall. Extremely premature babies may suffer from bleeding into the brain (intraventricular hemorrhage), sepsis, and other complications of their immature systems, including neurological and developmental damage. In survivors, bronchopulmonary dysplasia (a chronic scarring lung disease marked by prolonged oxygen need) may develop due to oxygen toxicity and mechanical ventilation. These complications are related to the severity of the disease, birth weight, and gestational age of the infant. Smaller babies are at greater risk of developing bronchopulmonary dysplasia.

How is it prevented, treated, and managed?

Prevention, treatment, prognosis

By far the biggest risk factor for respiratory distress syndrome (RDS) is prematurity. Preventing premature births could nearly eliminate RDS. Several causes of premature birth are preventable by good prenatal care. If the birth cannot be delayed beyond 34 weeks, the mother may be given corticosteroid therapy before birth, which accelerates fetal lung maturation. High-risk and premature infants require prompt attention by a pediatric resuscitation team. Healthcare providers

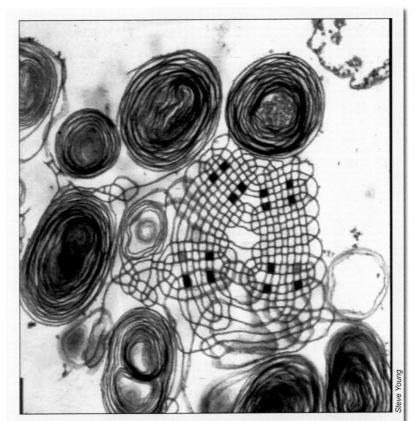

Without surfactant, breathing is impossible. Important basic science research led to the creation of surfactant replacement therapies that have dramatically improved survival of premature babies. However, there are still many mysteries about surfactant, including the function of this beautiful lattice-like structure; the colors were added to the squares of the lattice to help scientists understand how the lattices might form and work.

Steve Young

may deliver the baby and administer surfactant down the infant airways, either as soon as the premature baby is born or when RDS is diagnosed. The babies can be given respiratory support by mechanical ventilators with continuous positive airway pressure (CPAP) designed to prevent the alveoli from collapsing.

The use of oxygen has improved the life of many persons with respiratory disease. In the 1950s, however, its harmful effects were manifest when blindness occurred in premature infants given pure oxygen. As mechanical ventilation and critical care became more sophisticated in the 1960s and 1970s, neonatal intensive care unit beds became filled with RDS survivors. Although these premature infants could be kept alive longer on ventilators, many still died, and those who lived often developed bronchopulmonary dysplasia.

One of the greatest breakthroughs in the fight against lung disease was the development of surfactant replacement therapy, which saves these premature infants from an almost certain death. Its use has led to a dramatic decrease in mortality from nearly 100 percent to less than 10 percent. Typically, infants are able to breathe more easily within a few hours of receiving surfactant, and complications such as lung rupture are less likely to occur. There is a risk of bleeding into the lungs from surfactant treatment, especially in extremely low birth weight infants (those weighing less than 1,000 grams).

In addition, inhaled nitric oxide can improve oxygenation and reduce pulmonary inflammation. When begun soon after birth in these premature infants, nitric oxide administration improves the acute disease and also reduces the chance of chronic lung disease. As with most drugs, it can also have side effects, including an increased risk of bleeding.

Are we making a difference?

Research past, present, and future

Although earlier research defined the disease, the major breakthrough came with the discovery that lack of surfactant was the main defect. Studying the physiology of lungs under different conditions showed how critical surfactant was for breathing. Further research into the production, function, and composition of surfactant produced a deeper understanding of respiratory distress syndrome (RDS). The race was then on to develop surfactant replacement therapy. Both synthetic and animal-derived substances as well as components of surfactant were investigated as possible therapies. By 1987, clinical studies with surfactant therapy had begun in Japan, and studies in animal models of RDS were under way in the United States. The use of surfactant derived from calf lung produced gratifying results when given immediately after birth. There were concerns that disease transmission could occur from treating newborns with an animal-derived product, but fortunately this has not been reported.

Currently, all of the surfactant replacement therapies in use in the United States are animal derived. The surfactant replacement material is not as

Chronic lung disease by birth weight

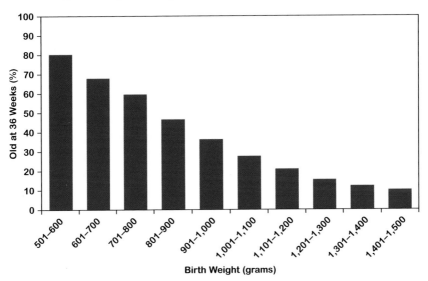

Incidence of bronchopulmonary dysplasia (BPD), defined as oxygen use at 36 weeks corrected postnatal age in premature babies. Horbar JD, Carpenter JH, Kenny M, eds. Vermont Oxford Network 2002 Very Low Birth Weight Database Summary. Burlington, VT: Vermont Oxford Network; 2003.

complete as natural human surfactant, and it is not effective in treating the type of RDS caused by the genetic mutation in SP-B, but for most cases, it has been wonderfully successful.

Despite the success of surfactant replacement in improving survival of premature babies with RDS, 5,000 to 10,000 newborns still develop bronchopulmonary dysplasia or other forms of chronic lung disease. The problem is most severe for the smallest babies in the extremely low birth weight group (500 to 699 grams), up to 85 percent of whom develop this complication. Preterm infants with bronchopulmonary dysplasia are at increased risk of death, re-hospitalization, and chronic and acute respiratory symptoms requiring therapy as compared with full-term infants. Therefore, recent research, both basic and clinical, has focused on efforts to prevent this complication. Clinical trials testing the usefulness of continuous nitric oxide inhalation therapy after birth and of repeated doses of surfactant to reduce the incidence and severity of bronchopulmonary dysplasia are ongoing.

Although there has been great reduction in the mortality and morbidity from RDS, the disease itself continues to increase with the rising rates of premature births. Strategies, such as giving continuous positive airway pressure (CPAP), ventilating babies without intubation, and nitric oxide therapy without mechanical ventilation, are being tested to prevent complications of RDS.

Nutrition is important for normal lung development and maturation. Several studies have shown that poor nutrition (specifically, a lack of protein) after birth may increase risk of lung injury that can lead to bronchopulmonary dysplasia. Vitamin A, a nutrient important for cell growth, has been shown to decrease bronchopulmonary dysplasia in some studies. Other nutrients may provide premature infants with added protection against this condition.

Surfactant therapy and other medical and critical care advances have increased survival among extremely low birth weight infants. These advances have presented additional challenges because these extremely premature babies often survive with residual long-term complications of RDS. If complications during pregnancy indicate that a premature birth is likely, obstetricians can test the amniotic fluid for surfactant in order to track fetal lung development. Several tests are available that correlate with the production of surfactant.

What we need to cure or eliminate respiratory distress syndrome of the newborn

Respiratory distress syndrome (RDS) can be cured but not eliminated. The defect has been discovered. A treatment has been developed, and thousands of lives have been saved. Despite this, newborns still develop bronchopulmonary dysplasia. Part of the problem is that surfactant replacement therapy and other medical and critical care advances have allowed the survival of extremely premature infants, who may later have residual long-term complications of RDS. Preventing prematurity is probably now the most important factor in eliminating RDS. Understanding of and advancements in nutrition and the delivery of critical care medicine to newborns will also improve the outcome of those with this condition.

References

1. Rodriguez RJ, Martin RJ, Fanaroff AA. Respiratory distress syndrome and its management. In: Fanaroff AA, Martin RJ, eds. *Fanaroff and Martin's Neonatal-Perinatal Medicine: Diseases of the Fetus and Infant.* 7th ed. St. Louis, MO: Mosby; 2002:1001–1011.
2. Goldenberg RL, Culhane JF, Iams JD, Romero R. Epidemiology and causes of preterm birth. *Lancet* 2008;371:75–84.
3. National Heart, Lung, and Blood Institute Web site. What is respiratory distress syndrome? Available at: http://www.nhlbi.nih.gov/health/dci/Diseases/rds/rds_all.html. Accessed January 21, 2010.
4. Robertson PA, Sniderman SH, Laros RK Jr, Cowan R, Heilbron D, Goldenberg RL, Iams JD, Creasy RK. Neonatal morbidity according to gestational age and birth weight from five tertiary care centers in the United States, 1983 through 1986. *Am J Obstet Gynecol* 1992;166:1629–1641.
5. Angus DC, Linde-Zwirble WT, Clermont G, Griffin MF, Clark RH. Epidemiology of neonatal respiratory failure in the United States: projections from California and New York. *Am J Respir Crit Care Med* 2001;164:1154–1160.
6. Centers for Disease Control and Prevention Web site. National Center for Health Statistics. Available at: http://www.cdc.gov/nchs. Accessed January 21, 2010.
7. American Lung Association Web site. Available at: http://www.lungusa.org. Accessed January 21, 2010.
8. March of Dimes Web site. Premature birth. Available at: http://www.marchofdimes.com/21209_11560.asp. Accessed January 21, 2010.
9. Halliday HL. Surfactants: past, present and future. *J Perinatol* 2008;28:S47–S56.
10. Nkadi PO, Merritt TA, Pillers DA. An overview of pulmonary surfactant in the neonate: genetics, metabolism, and the role of surfactant in health and disease. *Mol Genet Metab* 2009;97:95–101.

Web sites of interest

National Heart, Lung, and Blood Institute
Diseases and Conditions Index
www.nhlbi.nih.gov/health/dci/Diseases/rds/rds_all.html

Centers for Disease Control and Prevention
National Center for Health Statistics
www.cdc.gov/nchs

American Lung Association
www.lungusa.org

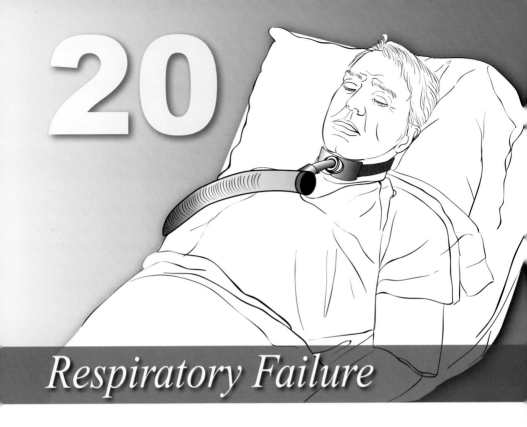

20

Respiratory Failure

Respiratory failure is not a disease *per se* but a consequence of the problems that interfere with the ability to breathe. The term refers to the inability to perform adequately the fundamental functions of respiration: to deliver oxygen to the blood and to eliminate carbon dioxide from it.

Respiratory failure has many causes and can come on abruptly (acute respiratory failure)—when the underlying cause progresses rapidly—or slowly (chronic respiratory failure)—when it is associated over months or even years with a progressive underlying process. Typically, respiratory failure initially affects the ability either to take up oxygen (referred to as *oxygenation failure*) or to eliminate carbon dioxide (referred to as *ventilatory failure*). Eventually, both functions cease when the respiratory failure becomes severe enough. This chapter will focus mainly on ventilatory failure; oxygenation failure is discussed in more detail in Chapter 2, which examines the acute respiratory distress syndrome (ARDS).

Whom does it affect?

Epidemiology, prevalence, and economic burden

Because so many underlying causes contribute to it, respiratory failure is a common and major cause of illness and death. It is the main cause of death from pneumonia and chronic obstructive pulmonary disease (COPD), which together comprise the third-leading cause of death in the United States today. It is also the main cause of death in many neuromuscular diseases, such as Lou Gehrig disease (amyotrophic lateral sclerosis or ALS), because these diseases weaken the respiratory muscles, rendering them incapable of sustaining breathing. Epidemiologic studies suggest that respiratory failure will become more common as the population ages, increasing by as much as 80 percent in the next 20 years (1).

Because respiratory failure is such a common cause of illness and death, the cost to society in terms of lost productivity and shortened lives is enormous. However, it is hard to quantify because the cause of death is more likely to be listed as pneumonia, COPD, or another underlying condition, rather than respiratory failure.

What are we learning about this disease?

Pathophysiology, causes: genetic, environment, microbes

In patients with neuromuscular disease, breathing first becomes a problem during sleep, when breathing normally slows and the weak respiratory muscles cannot keep up with the need to eliminate carbon dioxide. The rising carbon dioxide affects the acid–base balance of the body, and, in extreme cases, it could cause coma or even death.

Types of respiratory failure

Type		Typical Causes
Acute	Ventilatory	Drug overdose
	Oxygenation	Pneumonia
Chronic	Ventilatory	Neuromuscular disease
	Oxygenation	Pulmonary fibrosis

CASE STUDY

A 63-year-old lawyer complained of increasing fatigue and sleepiness over several months. He became short of breath when walking but had no problem breathing at rest. He did not feel rested when he awoke in the morning and often had morning headaches. When he was five years old, he had polio and was treated with an iron lung. A physical examination showed that his chest wall movement was diminished. He had severe curvature of the spine, and his abdomen did not rise during inspiration, which indicated a weak diaphragm. His pulmonary function (breathing) tests showed a sharply reduced lung volume and an inability to sustain a maximal breathing effort. His blood carbon dioxide was high and his oxygen low. A sleep study showed that his breathing slowed down even more at night, which was associated with a severe decrease in his oxygen level. He was prescribed a ventilator to use when he slept that delivered pressurized air to his lungs via a mask strapped over his nose and mouth. His sleep improved and his morning headaches went away, but he still became short of breath when he walked fast.

Comment

This scenario is typical of patients who develop chronic respiratory failure in the face of a slowly progressive neuromuscular condition. Despite the bout with polio 58 years earlier, the patient had been able to function normally until the aging process deteriorated his remaining motor nerves to the point where he could no longer sustain a normal level of breathing. Because the condition occurred so insidiously, his body had time to adapt and rendered him unaware of any breathing difficulty at rest. Shortness of breath at rest is a much bigger problem when respiratory failure is acute, such as that brought on by an asthma attack, pneumonia, or ARDS. Morning headaches are common because the rise in carbon dioxide at night causes a reflex widening of blood vessels in the brain, increasing the pressure of the fluid bathing the brain.

Many other causes besides respiratory muscle weakness contribute to respiratory failure (2). The ability to sustain normal respiration depends on the integration of many systems that are involved in breathing. Disruption of any one or a combination of these systems can induce failure. The respiratory center, located at the base of the brain, regulates breathing and determines how often and deeply we breathe. Depressed function of the respiratory center can con-tribute to respiratory failure. This condition is most often related to drugs, like narcotics, that blunt respiratory drive. Inadequate respiratory drive can also be inherited or acquired as a consequence of processes that damage neurons, such as strokes, severe trauma, or tumors, but this cause is rare.

The signal to breathe is carried to the muscles via nerves that can be para-lyzed abruptly by conditions such as the autoimmune Guillain–Barré syndrome or an overwhelming infection throughout the body, such as sepsis (see Chap-ter 22); less rapidly by conditions like ALS; or, as in the case of the patient previ-ously described, very slowly by post-polio syndrome and other conditions. High spinal cord injury, such as that suffered by the actor Christopher Reeves, causes respiratory failure because all muscles below the level of the injury are para-lyzed, including the respiratory muscles. Interestingly, patients with low neck fractures can still breathe because the nerves supplying the diaphragm arise from the mid-neck.

The nerve signal is then conveyed to the muscles via the myoneural junction. Antibodies to elements of the myoneural junction can cause severe weakness or paralysis, a chronic disease called *myasthenia gravis*. A spectrum of diseases affect the muscles themselves, including muscular dystrophy or acquired illnesses like polymyositis, in which the body's immune defense mechanisms attack the muscles, causing inflammation and weakness. All these conditions impair the abil-ity to move air in and out.

How is it prevented, treated, and managed?

Prevention, treatment, staying healthy, prognosis

The first principle in managing patients at risk for respiratory failure is to prevent progression of the underlying disease. Obviously, smoking cessation is an extremely important component of preventive therapy, as are influenza and pneu-mococcal vaccines. Pneumonia and asthma, for example, have specific therapies that include antibiotics and bronchodilators that should be instituted promptly.

Simultaneously, the respiratory failure must be addressed. If it is acute and severe, it is a medical emergency. Oxygen levels must be normalized as quickly as possible by providing supplemental oxygen. Patients with high carbon diox-ide levels need ventilatory support, so they receive pressurized gas from devices (ventilators) that increase pressure when triggered by the patient's inspiratory

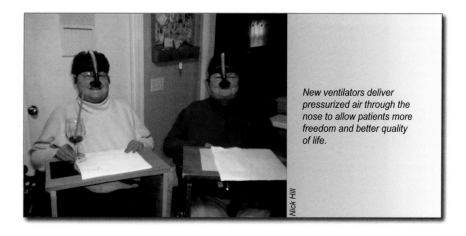

New ventilators deliver pressurized air through the nose to allow patients more freedom and better quality of life.

Nick Hill

effort or by a timer. The pressurized gas can be delivered via a plastic tube inserted into the trachea (invasive ventilation) or via a mask strapped over the nose and mouth or just the nose (noninvasive ventilation). Some patients may be given noninvasive ventilation only at night. This treatment allows a better quality of sleep so that symptoms of fatigue and daytime somnolence resolve.

Not all respiratory failure has a dire outlook. People may live functional lives at home for many years with chronic respiratory failure, and patients with acute respiratory failure can be ventilated until the acute disease is successfully treated. They may then return to a normal life. Nevertheless, all respiratory failure is serious and has potential life-threatening consequences.

Are we making a difference?

Research past, present, and future

During the past few decades, clinical and scientific research has resulted in greater understanding of respiratory failure and improved treatment. The iron lung, which assisted breathing by inducing an intermittent negative pressure around the body, was developed to cope with the respiratory failure that accompanied the polio epidemic in the 1950s. As intensive care units were developed to treat patients with acute respiratory failure during the 1960s, positive pressure ventilators that forced gas into endotracheal tubes became popular. Ventilators became increasingly sophisticated to enable patients to

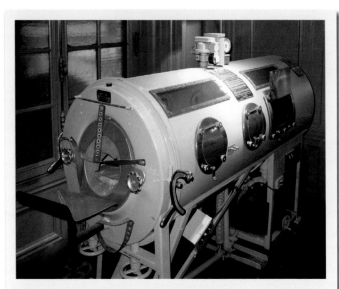

"Iron lungs" were the first ventilators used on a wide basis for the polio epidemic in the 1950s. They created an intermittent negative pressure around the chest so the lungs would expand and breathe.

"trigger" breaths so that they synchronized with the patient's own breathing pattern to enhance effectiveness and comfort. Over the past 15 years, better ventilators, better delivery of air to patients, and noninvasive ventilation have improved outcomes (3). Techniques to wean patients from invasive ventilation more quickly and safely have also been developed, cutting down on complications and costs in intensive care units (4).

Noninvasive ventilation has been an important advance in the treatment of acute respiratory failure. It reduces airway injury and the risk of pneumonia that occurs because bacteria otherwise track into the lungs through the endotracheal tube. It must, however, be used selectively, mainly for patients with COPD or heart failure. In heart failure, blood cannot be pumped adequately, causing fluid to back up in the lungs and interfere with oxygenation (pulmonary edema). Often, noninvasive ventilation can support the patient until the excess fluid is removed (3). Noninvasive ventilation has also been an important advance for patients with chronic respiratory failure, such as the patient described in the case study (5). It has also led to an appreciation of the important role that abnormal breathing during sleep plays in the progression of the respiratory failure (6). For patients with chronic respiratory failure, noninvasive ventilation is much easier and less expensive to administer than invasive ventilation, which requires a tube to be placed surgically into the trachea but often enables patients to live at home rather than in a long-term care institution.

Ways that breathing can fail

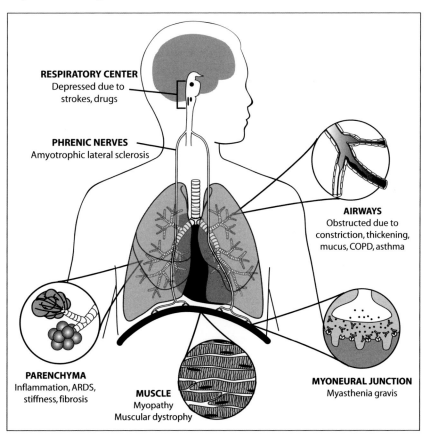

Several possible defects contribute to respiratory failure. The signal to breathe originates in the respiratory center and is sent by nerves via the myoneural junction to the respiratory muscles (such as the diaphragm). Respiratory function also depends on the integrity of the airways, lung structure, and blood vessels within the lungs. A few examples of diseases arising from the different defects are listed.

What we need to cure or eliminate respiratory failure?

Because respiratory failure is the consequence of many other primary conditions, its cure or elimination depends on more effective therapies for the primary conditions. For example, as treatments improve for the therapy of ARDS, pneumonia or ALS, respiratory failure as a consequence of these illnesses will diminish. The most significant recent advances in treating respiratory failure have been related to techniques and technology and future advances will occur in these areas. Ventilators are being developed with improved monitoring and other technological advances to reduce complications and enhance safety. New machines will synchronize better with patients, making them more comfortable. For long-term applications, machines are becoming more portable and quiet. In the future, small ventilators could even be strapped to a patient's belt, enabling ventilatory assistance while the patient walks in a mall or climbs stairs at home.

References

1. Carson SS, Cox CE, Holmes GM, Howard A, Carey TS. The changing epidemiology of mechanical ventilation: a population-based study. *J Intensive Care Med* 2006;21:173–182.
2. Mason R, Broaddus V, Murray J, Nadel J, eds. *Murray & Nadel's Textbook of Respiratory Medicine*. 4th edition. Amsterdam, The Netherlands: Elsevier Health Sciences; 2005. Chapters 85 and 86.
3. Nava S, Hill N. Non-invasive ventilation for acute respiratory failure. *Lancet* 2009; 374:250–259.
4. Girard TD, Ely EW. Protocol-driven ventilator weaning: reviewing the evidence. *Clin Chest Med* 2008;29:241–252.
5. Ozsancak A, D'Ambrosio C, Hill NS. Nocturnal noninvasive ventilation. *Chest* 2008;133:1275–1286.
6. Perrin C, D'Ambrosio C, White A, Hill NS. Sleep in restrictive and neuromuscular respiratory disorders. *Semin Respir Crit Care Med* 2005;26:117–130.

Web sites of interest

International Ventilator Users Network
www.ventusers.org

Post-Polio Health International
www.post-polio.org

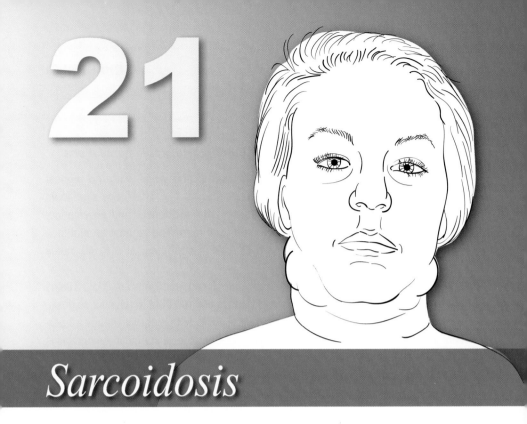

Sarcoidosis

Sarcoidosis is an inflammatory disease that can affect any organ and involves the lungs in 90 percent of patients. The tissue biopsy of patients with sarcoidosis has a characteristic appearance under the microscope consisting of clumps of specific types of inflammatory cells, called *granulomas*. Granulomas are an immune response to foreign particles that enter the body, which is why sarcoidosis is thought to have an environmental cause.

Sarcoidosis may exist without symptoms but is often discovered during a routine checkup. Usually, sarcoidosis is detected by a chest radiograph (x-ray) or chest computed tomography (CT) scan, which most commonly shows enlarged lymph nodes. The disease can last just one or two years and require minimal or no treatment, or it can span decades and require interventions. The symptoms depend on which organs the disease affects. The chronic progressive form of the disease involving the lungs results in shortness of breath and decline in overall quality of life. Patients with neurologic or heart involvement have the poorest outcome.

Whom does it affect?

Epidemiology, prevalence, economic burden, vulnerable populations

Sarcoidosis affects people of all ages throughout the world, with the highest incidence in those between the ages of 20 and 40 (1). There are significant racial and gender differences in disease severity, incidence, and prevalence. Worldwide, women are more often affected than men. The highest annual incidence has been observed in northern European countries, at 5 to 40 cases per 100,000 people per year (2).

With 36 cases per 100,000 people per year, African Americans are about 3 times more likely than Caucasian Americans (11 cases per 100,000) to have sarcoidosis. African American women are the most commonly affected group, with nearly a 3 percent lifetime risk for developing sarcoidosis (1). Sarcoidosis in African Americans is also more likely to be chronic, involve several organs, and lead to death (3).

No data on the economic burden due to sarcoidosis are available. Fatigue, joint pain, and shortness of breath can lead to lost work days and necessitate transfer to a less physically demanding job. Sarcoidosis accounts for less than 1 percent of hospital admissions in the United States (4).

Exposure to inorganic particles, insecticides, and moldy environments has been reported to be associated with sarcoidosis. Occupational studies

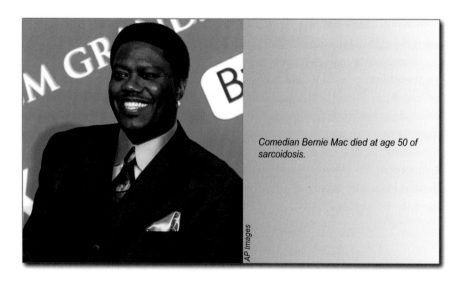

Comedian Bernie Mac died at age 50 of sarcoidosis.

AP Images

Incidence of sarcoidosis by age, race, and gender in Detroit, Michigan

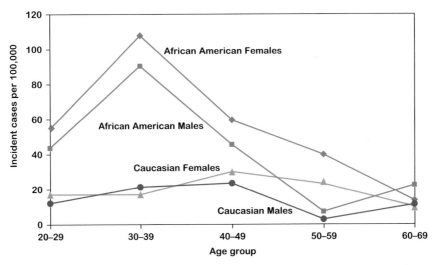

The incidence of sarcoidosis among Caucasian and African American men and women by age in a health maintenance organization in Detroit, Michigan, 1990–1994. Benjamin A. Rybicki, et al. Racial Differences in Sarcoidosis Incidence: A 5-Year Study in a Health Maintenance Organization, American Journal of Epidemiology, 1 February 1997, 145, 3, by permission of Oxford University Press.

have shown positive associations with metalworking, firefighting, service in the U.S. Navy, and handling of building supplies. Investigators have reported an increased incidence of sarcoidosis among New York City Fire Department rescue workers involved in the World Trade Center attacks of September 11, 2001. Socioeconomic status does not affect the risk of sarcoidosis, but low income and other financial barriers to care are associated with more severe sarcoidosis (5).

Susceptibility to sarcoidosis depends on an interaction between inherited genes and environmental exposures. Relatives of sarcoidosis patients are at higher risk of developing sarcoidosis compared to the general population. However, while family members are at higher risk, less than 1 percent of first- and second-degree relatives of sarcoidosis patients develop sarcoidosis (6). Sarcoidosis is not transmissible, and cigarette smokers are not at increased risk of developing sarcoidosis.

CASE STUDY

A 36-year-old woman sought medical evaluation for cough and shortness of breath that progressed over six months. She was diagnosed with bronchitis and given two courses of antibiotics. Her cough and shortness of breath persisted, and she was then diagnosed with asthma and was prescribed inhalers. She noted some improvement but then began feeling fatigued and experienced excessive sweating at night to the point that her bedclothes and bed sheets became wet. She lost 15 pounds over three months. She developed chest pain and discomfort in her hands and feet.

A chest radiograph showed large lymph nodes. Concerns were raised that she might have lymphoma or cancer. She was referred to a thoracic surgeon, who suspected sarcoidosis and referred her to a pulmonologist. The pulmonologist confirmed the diagnosis after taking tissue samples from the lung with a bronchoscope. The patient also completed pulmonary function tests that were normal. Because her symptoms interfered with her daily activities, she was prescribed prednisone, an anti-inflammatory steroid. By the time of her follow-up visit two months later, she had marked improvement in her symptoms.

Comment

The diagnosis of sarcoidosis can be difficult because there is no unique feature of the disease and no definitive test. It can be confused with chronic infections or other conditions that cause swollen lymph glands. Other diagnoses must be excluded before the diagnosis of sarcoidosis can be made. Characteristic x-ray images and a biopsy are usually required. Fortunately, bronchoscopy can usually obtain adequate tissue so that more invasive surgical biopsy is unnecessary. Prednisone used judiciously can markedly improve symptoms.

What are we learning about sarcoidosis?

Pathophysiology, causes: genetic, environment, microbes

Sarcoidal granulomas may spontaneously resolve or they may accumulate and persist. Accumulation and persistence of granulomas within an organ can lead to dysfunction and cause scarring. The extent and location of the granulomatous

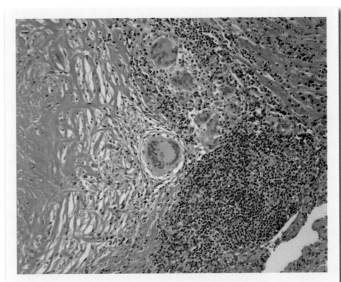

Granulomas are cellular reactions in which macrophages typically fuse together to form giant cells, and other inflammatory cells occupy specific areas of the lesion. The same reaction is seen in the lung with certain infections and inhaled particles.

inflammation determine the severity. For example, a large accumulation of granulomas within lymph nodes generally has little consequence, but minimal accumulation in the electrical conduction system of the heart can lead to sudden death.

Pulmonary fibrosis (scarring in the lung) occurs in 20 to 25 percent of patients, and can, in turn, lead to respiratory failure (7). Why fibrosis occurs in some individuals and not others is not known.

Several lines of thought have raised the suspicion that infectious agents or noninfectious particles cause sarcoidosis. Infectious agents, such as fungi and mycobacteria, and noninfectious particles, such as certain dusts, cause granulomatous reactions. Because sarcoidosis most commonly involves the lungs, followed by the eyes and skin, exposure to airborne agents in susceptible individuals has been suspected as the cause. The concept is supported by a higher incidence of cases in the spring and summer months when different infections peak. However, no infectious agent has been identified. Since sarcoidosis occurs worldwide and in all climates, it is likely that it is the cumulative result of immune responses to various environmental triggers, rather than to a single agent. Those who develop sarcoidosis likely inherit a tendency to respond more intensely to the inhaled agent.

How is it prevented, treated, and managed?

Prevention, treatment, staying healthy, prognosis

Since the cause of sarcoidosis is unknown, no way to prevent it exists. Studies show family members are at increased risk for developing sarcoidosis compared to the general population. However, the overall risk is extremely low; therefore, routine screening of family members should not be done.

Not all patients with sarcoidosis need treatment. In at least one third of patients, sarcoidosis resolves without treatment and causes no further problems. In fact, it is this spontaneous remission of sarcoidosis among individuals who participate in drug trials that confounds interpretation of results about the effectiveness of the drugs tested. Unfortunately, there are few large, well-designed sarcoidosis studies to guide treatment.

The decision to begin treatment is based on weighing the risks against the potential benefits. In general, treatment is begun for two reasons: 1) symptoms interfere with activities of daily living and cannot be controlled by simple

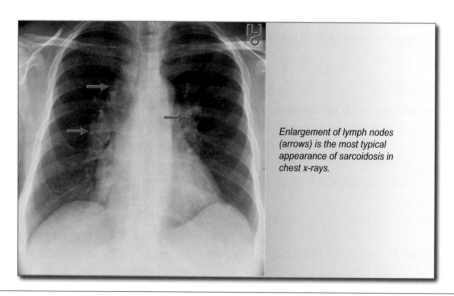

Enlargement of lymph nodes (arrows) is the most typical appearance of sarcoidosis in chest x-rays.

measures; and 2) organ function is threatened. When treatment is required, it is usually necessary to continue it for six months to a year, adjusting drug dosing according to response and to minimize side effects and complications.

Corticosteroids are the most effective treatment. Corticosteroids improve symptoms and lung function and probably prevent complications. For those who do not tolerate corticosteroids or when a combination approach is warranted, other agents might be used to reduce inflammation and prevent complications. Most published data on the use of non-corticosteroid agents are anecdotal and based on small studies.

Although sarcoidosis may result in periods of fatigue, body aches, joint pain, and respiratory symptoms such as cough and shortness of breath, for the vast majority, sarcoidosis is not permanently disabling. Several things can be done to remain healthy. Anyone who smokes should stop completely. Regular stretching exercises and exercises to promote cardiovascular health are recommended. Diet is particularly important for those on corticosteroids to minimize weight gain. Patients with active disease should have periodic follow-up visits with their physicians, which should include screening for eye and heart involvement.

Prognosis is variable and depends on gender, race, age, which organs are involved, the signs and symptoms at presentation, and which problems persist despite treatment. In the majority of patients, sarcoidosis improves or stabilizes in the first two years of illness. In nearly two thirds, spontaneous remission occurs within five years. Once the disease remits, it recurs in less than 5 percent of patients. Progressive sarcoidosis leads to death in less than 5 percent of cases (8). When it does, it is primarily due to progressive respiratory insufficiency or due to heart or neurologic involvement.

Are we making a difference?

Research past, present, and future

A great deal is known about the diagnosis, disease patterns, and clinical course of sarcoidosis. However, despite both a recent large, well-designed study funded by the National Heart, Lung, and Blood Institute called ACCESS and significant progress in methods to detect infectious agents, the cause of sarcoidosis remains unknown. Although the environmental trigger or triggers are yet to be identified, race and family history of disease are the most strongly identified risk factors, supporting the notion that a genetic susceptibility to sarcoidosis exists.

The risk for developing sarcoidosis has been associated with certain genes located on chromosome 6 that govern immune system function and are also involved in autoimmune disease and in rejection of transplanted organs. Technologic advances, including high-throughput techniques that allow sifting through the entire genome to identify disease genes, promise to define the cause of sarcoidosis. Significant progress has also been made in understanding the cellular interactions and the inflammatory proteins that are released that lead to granuloma formations. These studies have already helped direct novel treatment approaches. Well-designed clinical trials are now needed to determine their usefulness.

Investigators have reported that blood samples from patients with sarcoidosis often contain antibodies to proteins produced by mycobacteria, the bacteria that cause tuberculosis. Studies to verify the importance of mycobacterial infection as a cause of sarcoidosis are ongoing.

What we need to cure or eliminate sarcoidosis

Curing or eliminating sarcoidosis remains an elusive goal because its cause and how the disease develops are not known. Clinical trials of treatments may help in the management of these patients but real breakthroughs are likely to only occur after more is learned about the basics of this disease. Until the urgently needed research is carried out and yields answers, tens of thousands of Americans of all races will continue to suffer the burden of this disease.

References

1. Rybicki BA, Major M, Popovich J Jr, Maliarik MJ, Iannuzzi MC. Racial differences in sarcoidosis incidence: a 5-year study in a health maintenance organization. *Am J Epidemiol* 1997; 145:234–241.
2. Rybicki BA, Maliarik MJ, Major M, Popovich J Jr, Iannuzzi MC. Epidemiology, demographics, and genetics of sarcoidosis. *Semin Respir Infect* 1998;13:166–173.
3. Israel HL, Karlin P, Menduke H, DeLisser OG. Factors affecting outcome of sarcoidosis. Influence of race, extrathoracic involvement, and initial radiologic lung lesions. *Ann N Y Acad Sci* 1986;465:609–618.
4. Gorham ED, Garland CF, Garland FC, Kaiser K, Travis WD, Centeno JA. Trends and occupational associations in incidence of hospitalized pulmonary sarcoidosis and other lung diseases in Navy personnel: a 27-year historical prospective study, 1975–2001. *Chest* 2004;126:1431–1438.
5. Rabin DL, Thompson B, Brown KM, Judson MA, Huang X, Lackland DT, Knatterud GL, Yeager H Jr, Rose C, Steimel J. Sarcoidosis: social predictors of severity at presentation. *Eur Respir J* 2004;24:601–608.
6. Rybicki BA, Iannuzzi MC, Frederick MM, Thompson BW, Rossman MD, Bresnitz EA, Terrin ML, Moller DR, Barnard J, Baughman RP, et al. Familial aggregation of sarcoidosis. A case-control etiologic study of sarcoidosis (ACCESS). *Am J Respir Crit Care Med* 2001;164:2085–2091.
7. James DG. Life-threatening situations in sarcoidosis. *Sarcoidosis Vasc Diffuse Lung Dis* 1998;15:134–139.
8. Gideon NM, Mannino DM. Sarcoidosis mortality in the United States 1979–1991: an analysis of multiple-cause mortality data. *Am J Med* 1996;100:423–427.

Web sites of interest

National Heart, Lung, and Blood Institute
www.nhlbi.nih.gov/health/dci/Diseases/sarc/sar_whatis.html

Medline Plus
www.nlm.nih.gov/medlineplus/sarcoidosis.html

MedicineNet.com
www.medicinenet.com/sarcoidosis/article.htm

Foundation for Sarcoidosis Research
www.stopsarcoidosis.org

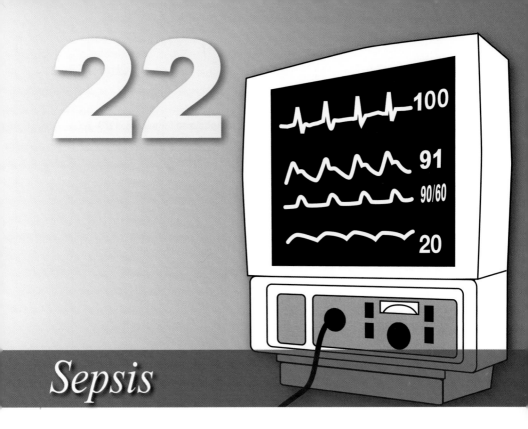

Sepsis

Sepsis or sepsis syndrome is a life-threatening medical condition characterized by an overwhelming infection and the body's inflammatory response to that infection. The source of the infection can be known, such as pneumonia, urinary tract infection, or skin or soft tissue infection, or unknown. Septic shock is a form of severe sepsis with associated low blood pressure that is life threatening. It leads to dysfunction of essentially all organs because of poor oxygenation and blood perfusion. With severe sepsis, failure of vital organs occurs, and the lungs are one of the most commonly affected organs. Sepsis is a common condition in the intensive care unit (ICU) and is associated with high mortality, morbidity, and cost.

Whom does it affect?

Epidemiology, prevalence, economic burden, vulnerable populations

The incidence of sepsis has increased considerably since the late 1970s. In 2000, the number of patients with a diagnosis of sepsis was approximately 660,000, increasing about 9 percent per year since 1979 (1). Sepsis accounts for 1 to 2 percent of all hospitalizations, and more than 50 percent of patients are

Overall in-hospital mortality rate among patients hospitalized for sepsis, 1979–2000

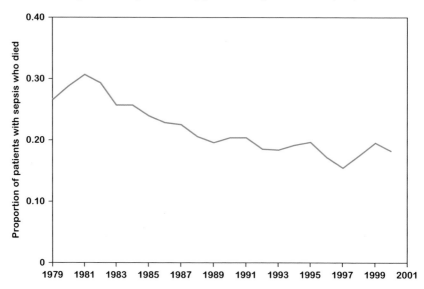

Mortality averaged 28 percent during the first six years of the study and 18 percent during the last six years (1). Copyright © 2005 Massachusetts Medical Society. All rights reserved.

cared for in an ICU (1,2). In response to improved supportive treatments and antibiotics, the in-hospital mortality rate has decreased over time to approximately 20 percent; however, the total number of deaths continues to increase, making sepsis the tenth-leading cause of death in the United States (1,3).

Sepsis also has significant associated morbidity and economic costs. Compared to the general population, survivors of sepsis reported poorer health-related quality of life and more physical dysfunction, including difficulty with work and activities of daily living (4,5). More than 30 percent of hospitalized sepsis survivors are not discharged to their homes. Instead, they are discharged to other care centers, such as nursing homes and rehabilitation facilities (1). In the United States, caring for patients with severe sepsis costs nearly $17 billion a year, with as much as $50,000 spent per patient (2).

Sepsis disproportionately affects the elderly and minority populations. The average age of those with the disease is reported to be in the early to mid-60s, and older age is an independent risk factor for death from sepsis (6). African Americans and other non-Caucasian minorities are consistently at an increased risk of developing

Sepsis

sepsis compared to Caucasians (1). In addition, African American men develop sepsis at a much younger age and are more likely to die from the condition.

What are we learning about this disease?

Pathophysiology, causes: genetic, environment, microbes

The cause of sepsis is not limited to bacterial infections, although they are the most common cause. Sepsis can also be caused by viral, fungal, and protozoan infections. Protein mediators (cytokines and chemokines) play a critical role in mobilizing the body's inflammatory response to contain and eradicate microbial infections.

Population-adjusted incidence of sepsis, according to race, 1979–2000

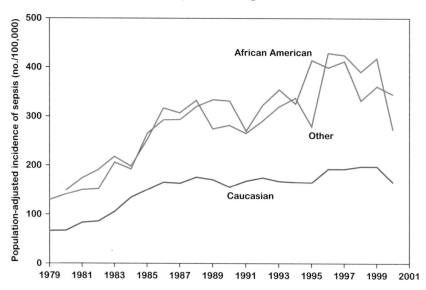

Points represent the annual incidence by race over two decades. Incidence and mortality are higher in minorities (1). Copyright © 2005 Massachusetts Medical Society. All rights reserved.

These cytokines and chemokines are chemical signals that trigger a wide-ranging cascade of events that change the metabolism and function of cells.

Inflammation enhances antimicrobial immunity; however, excessive inflammation results in "collateral damage" and causes vital organs to become dysfunctional, a characteristic feature of severe sepsis. Severe sepsis is the consequence of an exaggeration of the normal antimicrobial host defense mechanisms. One part of the body most affected by this exuberant inflammation are the blood vessels, which when injured become leaky. In the lungs, flooding of the airspace with inflammatory fluids disrupts the exchange of oxygen and carbon dioxide, resulting in acute respiratory distress syndrome (ARDS), a severe form of respiratory failure (see Chapter 2). A widespread increase in blood clotting in small blood vessels further disrupts normal blood flow and contributes to organ failure.

When the intense systemic inflammation begins to subside, the body attempts to repair the damaged organs. Through various mechanisms, the body inhibits the pro-inflammatory cytokines and chemokines. In the final stages of recovery, there is a process called *apoptosis*, or programmed cell death, during which inflammatory cells die and are harmlessly eliminated from tissues. This process, too, can be maladaptive because many of the mechanisms that halt inflammation also can affect immunity against infection by contributing to a condition referred to as *immunoparalysis,* in which beneficial inflammation is suppressed and a patient is at high risk for developing super-infections that are often difficult to treat.

How is it prevented, treated, and managed?

Prevention, treatment, staying healthy, prognosis

Prevention and early treatment of sepsis are of paramount importance. The best way to prevent sepsis is to prevent the inciting factor, which is infection that can

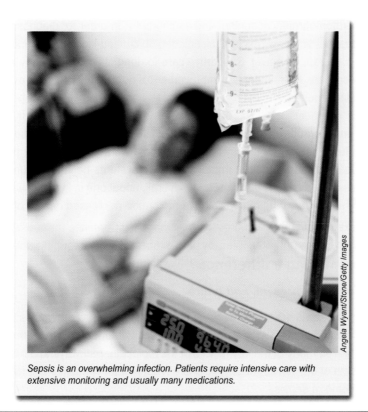

Sepsis is an overwhelming infection. Patients require intensive care with extensive monitoring and usually many medications.

Angela Wyant/Stone/Getty Images

occur in and out of the medical care setting. However, if appropriate antibiotics are given early in the course of an infection, the severity can be reduced and sepsis prevented. Controlling infection includes measures of personal hygiene such as hand washing and barrier protection in the hospital to prevent the transmission of disease via patient's body fluids. Those at increased risk should receive vaccinations for pneumococcus and influenza, common causes of respiratory infections.

The treatment of sepsis begins with a careful search for the underlying infectious cause with examination of the urine, sputum, spinal fluid, and blood for bacterial, viral, and fungal pathogens. Broad spectrum antibiotics are often given early, and these can be narrowed in spectrum once the causal organism is known. A major early concern is supporting circulation with intravenous fluids and medications that raise the blood pressure and improve blood flow and therefore increase the amount of oxygen supplied to vital organs and tissues. Patients with severe sepsis also may require advanced diagnostic studies, such as ultrasound, computed tomography scanning, and angiography, in order for diagnosis and to direct treatments for an infected gall bladder, obstructed kidneys, appendicitis, or ischemic or trapped bowel. Supportive care for lung failure and kidney failure is often necessary. Maintenance or improvement of nutritional status and avoidance of hospital-acquired infections and other ICU complications are also a priority.

The prognosis of sepsis is dependent on several factors, such as age, cause and duration of disease, and associated complications. Patients with chronic lung, heart, and kidney diseases have a worse prognosis for recovery. Many patients have impaired immune defense systems because of underlying diseases or medications that they take. Overall, about one in five sepsis patients die, and many survivors of sepsis have prolonged decreased quality of life and poor physical function.

Are we making a difference?

Research past, present, and future

There has been a great deal of new information about how molecules combine to cause both beneficial and harmful inflammation. Intense research efforts have characterized many of the key factors of the molecular pathways and have identified some of the individual genetic and environmental variability that influences the outcome of sepsis.

Proteins have been discovered that attach to a cell surface and send signals inside the cell. Secondary signaling molecules, such as nuclear factor kappa B (NF-κB) regulate DNA activity. NF-κB modifies synthesis of most of the inflammatory cytokines and chemokines (7). Another factor, Nrf-2, regulates many protective antioxidant and detoxifying proteins. A group of investigators has shown that a variation in the Nrf-2 gene can identify patients who are at increased risk for developing ARDS after major trauma. This could have important therapeutic implications (8).

Another group of investigators identified the role of a newly discovered protein, pre-B cell colony enhancing factor (PBEF), in generating inflammation and tissue injury (9). Measurement of blood levels of triggering receptor expressed on myeloid cells-2 (TREM-2), a molecule involved in the NF-κB pathway, seems to be highly sensitive and specific for distinguishing infectious from non-infectious causes of severe illness (10). It is likely that understanding of the molecules involved in the body's defense against infection and inflammation will allow future breakthroughs in treatment of severe sepsis.

Based on a multicenter randomized clinical trial (11), recombinant activated protein C, an anticoagulant, was approved by the U.S. Food and Drug Administration (FDA) for treatment of severe sepsis with multiple organ failure. This study showed a reduction in the death rate of severe sepsis from 30 to 25 percent. However, this treatment is not beneficial in patients with milder sepsis who have single organ failure and a lower risk of death (12), and it is not beneficial in treating young children (13). Furthermore, patients treated with recombinant activated protein C have an increased risk for serious bleeding complications (14), although complications can be minimized by appropriate patient selection criteria.

Although the anti-cytokine and other strategies that are based on understanding the molecular biology of sepsis have not had a noticeable influence on the treatment of severe sepsis, they have had a remarkable impact on the treatment of chronic inflammatory diseases, including inflammatory bowel disease, rheumatoid arthritis, and psoriasis.

What we need to cure or eliminate sepsis

Improved recognition, early organized approaches for the delivery of care, better antibiotics, improved nutrition and supportive care, and avoidance of ICU complications with newer technologies have had an enormous impact on improving outcome in severe sepsis over the decades. Further advances in these areas should continue to reduce the burden of sepsis. However, aging populations, increased prevalence of organ transplantation, more aggressive treatment of cancer, autoimmune diseases that increase susceptibility to infections, and limitations in early access to healthcare have contributed to the sustained high mortality of severe sepsis.

Research in sepsis aims to better understand the molecular networks in order to identify critical points that may be amenable to interventions and to learn why individuals with disease vary in their outcome. Discovery of markers that predispose some individuals to severe sepsis, that identify early sepsis, or that correlate with clinical outcome would help to better manage the disease and determine when intervention should take place. Translating this knowledge into treatment and cure of patients in the ICU will require large controlled clinical trials.

References

1. Martin GS, Mannino DM, Eaton S, Moss M. The epidemiology of sepsis in the United States from 1979 through 2000. *N Engl J Med* 2003;348:1546–1554.
2. Angus DC, Linde-Zwirble WT, Lidicker J, Clermont G, Carcillo J, Pinsky MR. Epidemiology of severe sepsis in the United States: analysis of incidence, outcome, and associated costs of care. *Crit Care Med* 2001;29:1303–1310.
3. National Center for Health Statistics. *Health, United States, 2007 With Chartbook on Trends in the Health of Americans.* Hyattsville, MD: US Department of Health and Human Services; 2007.
4. Heyland DK, Hopman W, Coo H, Tranmer J, McColl MA. Long-term health-related quality of life in survivors of sepsis. Short Form 36: a valid and reliable measure of health-related quality of life. *Crit Care Med* 2000;28:3599–3605.
5. Perl TM, Dvorak L, Hwang T, Wenzel RP. Long-term survival and function after suspected gram-negative sepsis. *JAMA* 1995;274:338–345.
6. Martin GS, Mannino DM, Moss M. The effect of age on the development and outcome of adult sepsis. *Crit Care Med* 2006;34:15–21.
7. Blackwell TS, Christman JW. The role of nuclear factor-kappa B in cytokine gene regulation. *Am J Respir Cell Mol Biol* 1997;17:3–9.
8. Marzec JM, Christie JD, Reddy SP, Jedlicka AE, Vuong H, Lanken PN, Aplenc R, Yamamoto T, Yamamoto M, Cho HY, et al. Functional polymorphisms in the transcription factor NRF2 in humans increase the risk of acute lung injury. *FASEB J* 2007;21:2237–2246.
9. Garcia JG. Searching for candidate genes in acute lung injury: SNPs, Chips and PBEF. *Trans Am Clin Climatol Assoc* 2005;116:205–219.
10. Klesney-Tait J, Turnbull IR, Colonna M. The TREM receptor family and signal integration. *Nat Immunol* 2006;7:1266–1273.
11. Bernard GR, Vincent JL, Laterre PF, LaRosa SP, Dhainaut JF, Lopez-Rodriguez A, Steingrub JS, Garber GE, Helterbrand JD, Ely EW, et al, for the Recombinant human protein C Worldwide Evaluation in Severe Sepsis (PROWESS) study group. Efficacy and safety of recombinant human activated protein C for severe sepsis. *N Engl J Med* 2001;344:699–709.
12. Abraham E, Laterre PF, Garg R, Levy H, Talwar D, Trzaskoma BL, François B, Guy JS, Brückmann M, Rea-Neto A, et al, for the Administration of Drotrecogin Alfa (Activated) in Early Stage Severe Sepsis (ADDRESS) Study Group. Drotrecogin alfa (activated) for adults with severe sepsis and a low risk of death. *N Engl J Med* 2005;353:1332–1341.
13. Nadel S, Goldstein B, Williams MD, Dalton H, Peters M, Macias WL, Abd-Allah SA, Levy H, Angle R, Wang D, et al, for the REsearching severe Sepsis and Organ dysfunction in children: a gLobal perspective (RESOLVE) study group. Drotrecogin alfa (activated) in children with severe sepsis: a multicentre phase III randomised controlled trial. *Lancet* 2007;369:836–843.
14. Vincent JL, Bernard GR, Beale R, Doig C, Putensen C, Dhainaut JF, Artigas A, Fumagalli R, Macias W, Wright T, et al. Drotrecogin alfa (activated) treatment in severe sepsis from the global open-label trial ENHANCE: further evidence for survival and safety and implications for early treatment. *Crit Care Med* 2005;33:2266–2277.

Web sites of interest

Medline Plus
Sepsis
www.nlm.nih.gov/medlineplus/sepsis.html

National Institute of General Medical Sciences
Sepsis Fact Sheet
www.nigms.nih.gov/Publications/factsheet_sepsis.htm

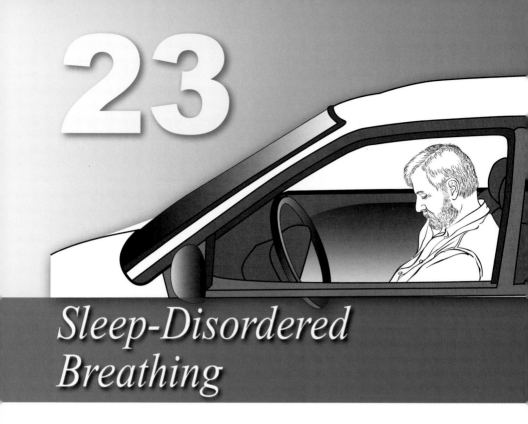

Sleep-Disordered Breathing

Sleep-disordered breathing is an umbrella term for several chronic conditions in which partial or complete cessation of breathing occurs many times throughout the night, resulting in daytime sleepiness or fatigue that interferes with a person's ability to function and reduces quality of life. Symptoms may include snoring, pauses in breathing described by bed partners, and disturbed sleep. Obstructive sleep apnea (OSA), which is by far the most common form of sleep-disordered breathing, is associated with many other adverse health consequences, including an increased risk of death (1–3).

To be properly diagnosed, patients with suspected sleep-disordered breathing must be evaluated by a polysomnogram (sleep test), which measures approximately a dozen physiologic parameters during sleep. One of the most important measurements is breathing and its cessation during sleep. A breathing pause of 10 seconds or more is termed an *apnea*. Not surprisingly, apneas may be associated with oxygen desaturation (a decrease in blood oxygen) and other bodily responses as the person struggles to breathe. These arousals may consist of flexing of muscles, including those of the airways, and change in the electrical activity of the brain as measured by an electroencephalogram (EEG). Arousals are complex phenomena that may involve discharges of brain chemicals of the adrenalin family, which may contribute to the health conditions associated with sleep apnea. Desaturation and arousals also occur with hypopnea (partial decrease in air flow). The apnea-hypopnea index is the number of apneas and hypopneas that occur per hour of sleep and is an important measure of the severity of sleep apnea, along with the depth of desaturation.

A single-night polysomnogram in a sleep laboratory can accurately diagnose sleep apnea in most patients. With portable equipment, the diagnosis of sleep apnea is possible in the home setting, and this approach may provide improved access to sleep apnea diagnostic testing.

Whom does it affect?

Epidemiology, prevalence, economic burden, vulnerable populations

Estimates of the prevalence of sleep-disordered breathing vary widely, depending on the methodology. Conservatively, based on laboratory or portable home tests, 4 percent of men, 2 percent of women, and 2 percent of children ages 8 to 11 in the United States have sleep-disordered breathing (4,5). Other surveys estimate that between 5 and 10 percent of the U.S. adult population have

Prevalence of sleep-disordered breathing among U.S. adults

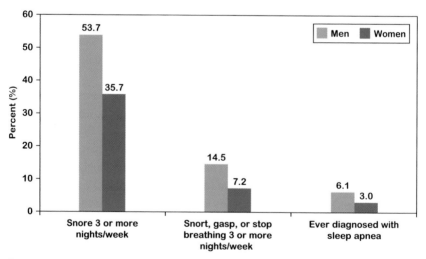

This survey shows how common sleep-disordered breathing problems are.
Unpublished data from the National Health and Nutrition Examination Survey, 2005–2006.

OSA (5–7); 7 percent have breathing pauses during sleep that put them at risk for more severe sleep events, and 23 to 59 percent snore (7–10). Unpublished data from a nationally representative sample of U.S. adults over age 20 show that the symptoms of sleep-disordered breathing (for example, snoring) are more likely to be reported by men than women. From 1980 to 1990, the number of office visits in the United States resulting in a diagnosis of sleep apnea increased from 108,000 to 1.3 million (11).

Despite the increased awareness of sleep-disordered breathing, it has been suggested that 93 percent of women and 82 percent of men with signs and symptoms of moderate to severe sleep-disordered breathing remain undiagnosed (6).

Factors that have been identified in studies to increase the risk of developing sleep apnea include obesity, male gender, and some ethnic groups (African American, Asian, and Native American) (12). Additional risk factors include

Sleep-disordered breathing and cardiovascular disease

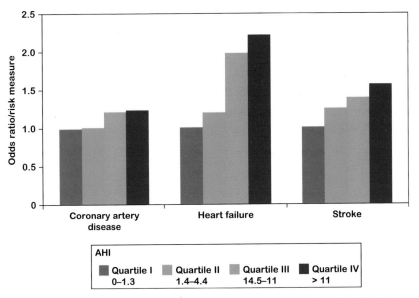

An early study of more than 6,400 patients with mild to moderate sleep-disordered breathing found an association between sleep-apnea severity as measured by the apnea-hypopnea index (AHI) and coronary artery disease, heart failure, and stroke. Those with the highest AHI were one-and-a-half times more likely to have had a stroke and more than twice as likely to have heart failure than those with lowest AHI, even when adjusted for other known risk factors, including age, sex, race, body size, hypertension, smoking, and cholesterol. Adapted from American Journal of Respiratory and Critical Care Medicine, Vol 163. pp 19-25, 2001.

CASE STUDY

William Howard Taft, the 27th President of the United States, and later the 10th Chief Justice, lived before sleep apnea was recognized as a disease, but throughout his life he exhibited the classic symptoms and signs (14). At the time of his inauguration at age 51, he weighed between 300 and 332 pounds and had a 19-inch neck. He had excessive daytime sleepiness and loud habitual snoring. In his fifties, Taft developed high blood pressure. He had limited exercise tolerance, and by his mid-sixties, he had signs of heart disease (angina) and breathlessness, which limited

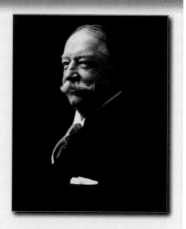

his activity. Toward the end of his presidency, he developed an irregular heart beat that is commonly associated with sleep apnea (atrial fibrillation). Taft lost a remarkable amount of weight (he slimmed down to about 250 pounds), which was associated with an improvement in his daytime sleepiness and blood pressure. It may have also increased his longevity. Taft was 72 when he died on March 8, 1930. A medical bulletin issued by the Supreme Court upon his resignation earlier in the year attributed his serious health condition to "general hardening of the arteries."

Comment

There are reports of President Taft falling asleep during important meetings and while serving as Chief Justice of the Supreme Court. To Taft, this was an embarrassment and a blow to his esteem and reputation. For other patients, however, it can have more serious consequences. To a truck driver, it could be deadly. Lack of adequate sleep at night for any reason leads to daytime somnolence, and habitual lack of restful sleep can lead to uncontrollable sleep attacks.

nasal obstruction; large tonsils (particularly in children); an underactive thyroid gland; the use of alcohol, tobacco, and sedatives; menopause in women; and higher levels of testosterone.

The economic burden of sleep-disordered breathing is significant (13). Sleep-disordered breathing adversely affects daytime alertness and cognition and has been linked to occupational and driving impairment. Sleep apnea has also been shown to increase healthcare utilization. In any assessment of the economic burden of sleep apnea, there are two important considerations: 1) it is highly prevalent in the middle-aged work force, and 2) it contributes to other chronic health conditions, such as heart disease and diabetes, and increases the risk of having a stroke and being in an accident at work or in the car.

What are we learning about sleep-disordered breathing?

Pathophysiology, causes: genetic, environment

No single cause of sleep apnea has been identified, although the associations with weight and neck size mentioned above are well known. Family history and genetic susceptibility studies show that a third of the total variability in sleep apnea severity in populations can be accounted for by heritability or genetic susceptibility (1,15). The bony and soft tissue structures of the face, as well as the heritability of obesity, are potential mechanisms by which genetics plays a role in sleep apnea.

The most common breathing disorder of sleep is OSA, which is characterized by recurrent narrowing or collapse of the back of the throat because of the loss of muscle tone that occurs during sleep (16). A less common form, central sleep apnea, is distinguished by cessation of breathing efforts during sleep. There is no struggle to breathe; the brain just does not send the proper breathing signals. Both result in repetitive events of insufficient air flow, oxygen absorption, and carbon dioxide exhalation. Reduction in blood oxygen levels may lead to a hormonal stress response by the body. This reaction may arouse, but not fully awaken, the sleeper, who repeats the events with the next period of sleep. If the cycle of arousals is repeated many times during the night, a cascade of stress-hormone release ensues, which is thought to be responsible for many of the adverse health consequences associated with sleep-disordered breathing.

The upper airway in patients with OSA is often smaller than normal. It may be narrowed by fat deposition in obese individuals or other structural factors, such as airway length, position of the jaw, or size of the tongue. A narrowed air passage can collapse more frequently and completely when the muscles of the throat, which keep the upper airway open during wakefulness, relax during

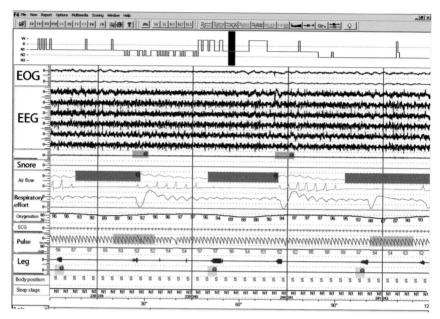

This sleep tracing typically records 16 different parameters simultaneously. The electroencephalogram (EEG) (brain waves) stages sleep. The electro-occulogram (EOG) records rapid eye movement, which is correlated with dreaming. Snoring, air flow, respiratory effort, oxygenation, electrocardiogram (ECG) findings, pulse, leg movement (leg), body position, and sleep stage are the other items assessed.

sleep. Changes in body position and the reduced lung expansion that occur with sleep interact with these other factors and may lead to further upper airway vulnerability.

Experimental animal studies as well as observations in patients with central sleep apnea show that the brain centers responsible for the control of rhythmic respiratory muscle activity are more unstable compared to people without this disorder (15). Some individuals may have both obstructive and central sleep apnea.

How is it prevented, treated, and managed?

Prevention, treatment, staying healthy, prognosis

A major problem is the lack of recognition of the disorder by both the patient and physician. This unawareness may lead to delayed diagnosis. Snoring and daytime fatigue or sleepiness are so common that they may not be recognized

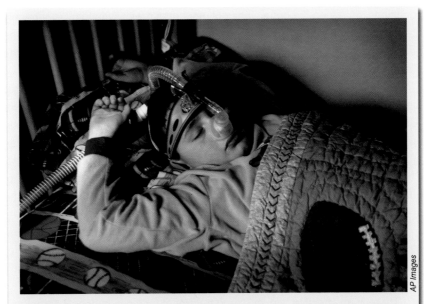

For children suffering from sleep apnea, surgical treatment with removal of tonsils (and adenoids) is the first choice. However, the long-term effects of this procedure on sleep-disordered breathing in these children are poorly understood.

as abnormal. There is considerable variation in the severity of sleep apnea from night to night, depending upon duration of sleep, body position, time spent in different stages of sleep, and other factors, such as alcohol consumption before going to bed. Alcohol and certain sleeping medications may cause deeper relaxation of the airways during sleep and a blunting of the sleeper's arousal response, thus allowing longer and more frequent apneas and greater desaturations.

Prevention of weight gain and obesity is critical for reducing the risk of developing clinically significant OSA. Appropriate evaluation and treatment of any nasal passage obstruction is important in reducing the collapsibility of the upper airway. Smoking cessation should be pursued by all patients. Avoiding alcohol and sedatives and developing better sleep hygiene may be helpful.

Physicians use the apnea-hypopnea index to assess the severity of sleep apnea based on the number of complete cessations of breathing (apnea) and partial obstructions (hypopnea). Although the apnea-hypopnea index is interpreted in the context of the patient's symptoms, age, and other medical conditions, an apnea-hypopnea index of more than 5 with symptoms is generally abnormal enough to warrant treatment. As the condition is usually chronic, in the absence of significant modification of a risk factor, the treatment prescribed should be used long term.

Treatments for OSA work by physically increasing the size of the upper airway. The most effective treatment is a continuous positive airway pressure (CPAP) device that delivers pressurized air to the upper airway, via a mask, splinting the airway open. However, the effectiveness of this treatment is often substantially reduced or nullified by inconsistent or inadequate use by patients. Professionally assisted adjustments of the mask size and type, the addition of humidity, and the treatment of nasal congestion and blockage may improve the ability to use this treatment.

For children suffering from sleep apnea, surgical treatment with removal of tonsils (and adenoids) is the first choice. However, the long-term effects of this procedure on sleep-disordered breathing in these children are poorly understood.

There is no effective and safe drug treatment for sleep apnea. External and intranasal dilators improve snoring, but their efficacy in reducing sleep-disordered breathing has not been adequately shown by controlled trials. In certain patients, surgical treatment or dental devices may be effective, but more studies are needed.

Are we making a difference?

Research past, present, and future

Although breathing abnormalities that occur during wakefulness and sleep have been reported since the 1800s, the high prevalence of disordered breathing that occurs only during sleep was not recognized until 1993 (4). The risk factors for sleep-disordered breathing and the high prevalence of sleep apnea, as well as the adverse health conditions associated with untreated sleep apnea, including increased mortality, have been identified by multiple large-scale observational studies. There is, however, an urgent need for large-scale clinical studies to determine the natural course and benefit of treatments on the longer-term health in people with all levels of sleep-disordered breathing, especially with regard to its severity, effect on cardiovascular health, and survival. Given the remarkable rise of obesity and the high prevalence of diabetes today, it would also be important to learn the effects of these conditions on the course and treatment of sleep apnea. Intervention at early stages has the potential to become an effective prevention strategy.

These studies should also assess the cost to society for sleep apnea and its treatment. Confirmation of whether portable and home-based diagnostic monitoring and auto-adjusting therapeutic CPAP devices could adequately supplement formal laboratory-based evaluation, and, if so, in which populations, would lead to more cost-effective healthcare delivery. Studies thus far support the use of oral appliances in mild to moderate sleep-disordered breathing and the use of surgery primarily as adjunctive treatment for adults or in "CPAP failures." Electrical stimulation of the nerves to activate the upper airway muscles and dilate the airway has been associated with beneficial effects on sleep-disordered breathing, but this approach needs further study to determine efficacy as well as the design of equipment for clinical use.

It is as yet not clear whether the candidate genes for sleep apnea (for example, the APOE epsilon gene) lead directly to sleep apnea or if these genes are linked to intermediate factors that increase the risk of sleep apnea via their effects on other factors, such as facial structure and obesity (15). Future studies involving analyses of multiple genes simultaneously in well-defined subgroups of persons with sleep apnea hold the promise for development of predictive models that will enable early diagnosis and intervention in the appropriate populations. A genetic approach also may lead to better understanding of the basic mechanisms of the condition, which is a prerequisite for the development of future therapies.

What we need to cure or eliminate sleep-disordered breathing

Elimination of sleep apnea remains a distant goal, as the current struggles are simply awareness, diagnosis, and management. Reducing obesity in the population would no doubt reduce sleep apnea. Safe and effective drugs may offer the best chance for reduction of sleep-disordered breathing, but finding these drugs will depend on a better understanding of the neurophysiology and biochemistry of sleep. This understanding could lead to as yet unanticipated fruitful interventions. Discoveries important to sleep-disordered breathing could come from other fields far removed from sleep.

References

1. Al Lawati NM, Patel SR, Ayas NT. Epidemiology, risk factors, and consequences of obstructive sleep apnea and short sleep duration. *Prog Cardiovasc Dis* 2009;51:285–293.
2. Caples SM, Garcia-Touchard A, Somers VK. Sleep-disordered breathing and cardiovascular risk. *Sleep* 2007;30:291–303.
3. Young T, Finn L, Peppard PE, Szklo-Coxe M, Austin D, Nieto FJ, Stubbs R, Hla KM. Sleep disordered breathing and mortality: eighteen-year follow-up of the Wisconsin sleep cohort. *Sleep* 2008;31:1071–1078.
4. Young T, Palta M, Dempsey J, Skatrud J, Weber S, Badr S. The occurrence of sleep-disordered breathing among middle-aged adults. *N Engl J Med* 1993;328:1230–1235.
5. Rosen CL, Larkin EK, Kirchner HL, Emancipator JL, Bivins SF, Surovec SA, Martin RJ, Redline S. Prevalence and risk factors for sleep-disordered breathing in 8- to 11-year-old children: association with race and prematurity. *J Pediatr* 2003;142:383–389.
6. Young T, Peppard PE, Gottlieb DJ. Epidemiology of obstructive sleep apnea: a population health perspective. *Am J Respir Crit Care Med* 2002;165:1217–1239.
7. Decker MJ, Lin JM, Tabassum H, Reeves WC. Hypersomnolence and sleep-related complaints in metropolitan, urban, and rural Georgia. *Am J Epidemiol* 2009;169:435–443.
8. Hiestand DM, Britz P, Goldman M, Phillips B. Prevalence of symptoms and risk of sleep apnea in the US population: results from the National Sleep Foundation Sleep in America 2005 poll. *Chest* 2006;130:780–786.
9. Nieto FJ, Young TB, Lind BK, Shahar E, Samet JM, Redline S, D'Agostino RB, Newman AB, Lebowitz MD, Pickering TG. Association of sleep-disordered breathing, sleep apnea, and hypertension in a large community-based study. Sleep Heart Health Study. *JAMA* 2000;283:1829–1836.
10. Foley D, Ancoli-Israel S, Britz P, Walsh J. Sleep disturbances and chronic disease in older adults: results of the 2003 National Sleep Foundation Sleep in America Survey. *J Psychosom Res* 2004;56:497–502.
11. Namen AM, Dunagan DP, Fleischer A, Tillett J, Barnett M, McCall WV, Haponik EF. Increased physician-reported sleep apnea: the National Ambulatory Medical Care Survey. *Chest* 2002;121:1741–1747.
12. Tischler PV, Larkin EK, Schluchter MD, Redline S. Incidence of sleep-disordered breathing in an urban adult population: the relative importance of risk factors in the development of sleep-disordered breathing. *JAMA* 2003;289:2230–2237.
13. AlGhanim N, Comondore VR, Fleetham J, Marra CA, Ayas NT. The economic impact of obstructive sleep apnea. *Lung* 2008;186:7–12.
14. Sotos JG. Taft and Pickwick: sleep apnea in the White House. *Chest* 2003;124:1133–1142.
15. Pack AI. Advances in sleep-disordered breathing. *Am J Respir Crit Care Med* 2006;173:7–15.
16. Eckert DJ, Malhotra A. Pathophysiology of adult obstructive sleep apnea. *Proc Am Thorac Soc* 2008;5:144–153.

Web sites of interest

American Academy of Sleep Medicine
www.aasmnet.org/PatientsPublic.aspx

American Sleep Apnea Association
www.sleepapnea.org

Centers for Disease Control and Prevention
Sleep and Sleep Disorders: A Public Health Challenge
www.cdc.gov/sleep

National Institutes of Health
National Center on Sleep Disorders Research
www.nhlbi.nih.gov/sleep

National Sleep Foundation
www.sleepfoundation.org

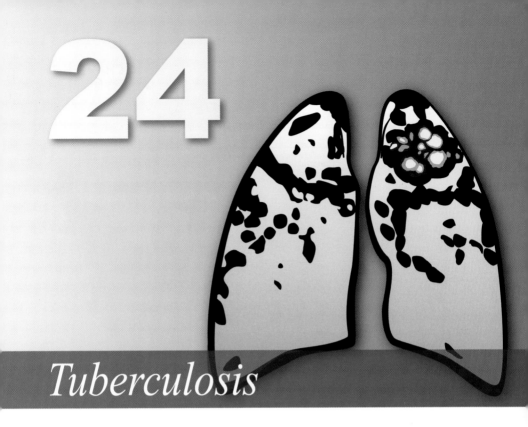

24

Tuberculosis

Tuberculosis (TB) is an infectious disease that is acquired by inhaling the bacteria that cause the disease. About 90 percent of those who become infected show no sign of disease (latent infection), but harbor the organism and have a risk of developing active TB later. Left untreated, a third to a half of those who do develop disease will die from it. The others with active disease will go into remission or have chronic symptoms. Those with active TB can infect others. Effective drugs have been available for more than half a century, and virtually all cases of TB should be curable, although the emergence of drug-resistant bacteria has made the treatment much longer, more difficult, and expensive.

Whom does it affect?

Epidemiology, prevalence, economic burden, vulnerable populations

TB is the greatest killer of people in recorded history. Lemuel Shattuck, who pioneered the use of statistics in public health, reported that between 1811 and 1820, nearly a quarter (23.4 percent) of all deaths in New York City occurred from TB. Sixty years later, Dr. Robert Koch, the German scientist who identified the TB bacterium, wrote "one-seventh of all human beings die of tuberculosis,

Rate* of TB cases, by state/area — United Sates, 2008†

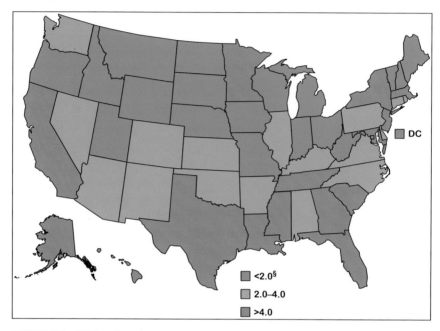

DC

<2.0§
2.0–4.0
>4.0

SOURCE: National TB Surveillance System.
* Per 100,000 population.
† Data updated as of February 18, 2009. Data for 2008 are provisional.
§ TB rate cutoff points were based on terciles: 18 states had TB case rates of <2.0 (range: 0.46–1.99) per 100,000, 17 states had TB case rates of 2.0–4.0 (range: 2.03–3.92) per 100,000, and 15 states and the District of Columbia had TB case rates of >4.0 (range: 4.02–9.63) per 100,000.

The number and rate of TB cases has steadily fallen, but the number of foreign-born persons with TB has remained constant.

and . . . if one considers only the productive middle-age groups, tuberculosis carries away one-third and often more of these . . ." (1).

Much of the history of modern medicine is tied to efforts to understand and curtail this remarkable killer whose exact nature eluded discovery until the mid-19th century, when it was discovered to be transmissible. Later, in 1882, it was shown to be caused by bacteria. Grassroots health efforts followed, producing sanatoria, public health organizations, and new government health departments. In the next decades, researchers developed diagnostic sputum and skin tests, as well as a TB vaccine. These advances, along with better understanding of the disease, reduced its prevalence. In 1944, the first antibiotic

Tuberculosis

Number and rate* of TB cases among U.S.- and foreign-born persons, by year reported—United States, 1993–2008†

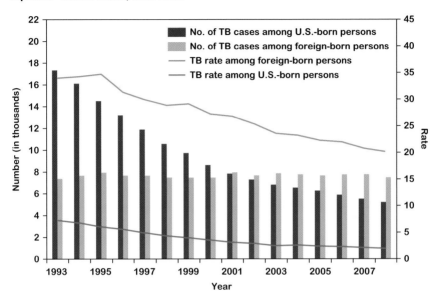

SOURCE: National TB Surveillance System.
* Per 100,000 population.
† Data are updated as of February 18, 2009. Data for 2008 are provisional.

for TB—streptomycin—was discovered, and by 1970, there were more than half a dozen effective drugs to treat TB. Unfortunately, these discoveries led to complacency and neglect on the part of the public and public health officials. As infection and mortality rates dropped, TB hospitals closed, and research and public health attention shifted to other areas. But in 1988, with human immunodeficiency virus (HIV) infection on the rise, the downward trend in TB reversed, and healthcare systems were unable to handle its resurgence. HIV attacks the cells responsible for mounting the primary immune defense and renders individuals susceptible to TB. Following decades of decline, TB rates in the United States began to rise again, until 1993, when the government increased support for all aspects of the war against TB. The incidence of disease again began to fall. In 2008, 12,898 new cases of TB were reported in the United States, for a rate of 4.2 per 100,000 people—the lowest ever recorded (2).

Beyond the United States, however, the number of TB cases continues to rise. In 2007, the World Health Organization estimated that there were 9.3 million

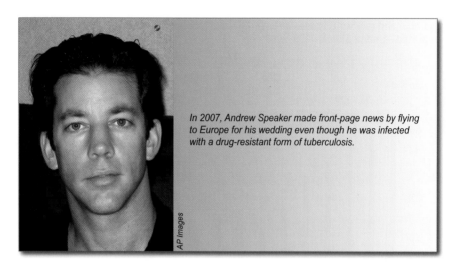

In 2007, Andrew Speaker made front-page news by flying to Europe for his wedding even though he was infected with a drug-resistant form of tuberculosis.

AP Images

new cases and 1.3 million deaths throughout the world each year (2). TB has been estimated to account for an annual loss of 8.7 million years of life worldwide (3). Furthermore, about a third of the world's population is believed to have latent infection (4). More than half of the persons developing TB in the United States are foreign born (2). It became apparent that TB control efforts in the United States and other low-prevalence countries must include global TB control as a keystone issue. In the 1990s, a large international effort to control TB began, resulting in more effective national TB control programs.

The enormous number of infections worldwide is not the only problem. Today, 20 percent of TB cases in the world are resistant to at least one drug used to treat the disease, and 5 percent of cases are multidrug resistant (MDR-TB), a much more serious condition in which the bacteria are resistant to the two main therapeutic agents, isoniazid and rifampin. Rates of resistance vary greatly between countries. Among new cases in the United States, 7 percent are resistant to isoniazid and 1.2 percent are resistant to isoniazid and rifampin and, thus, have MDR-TB. This rate is in contrast to that in countries such as Georgia, Uzbekistan, and Azerbaijan, where the resistance to one drug is about 50 percent. The number of MDR-TB cases is highest in India and China, but exact information about the prevalence of drug resistance is lacking because testing has not been available in much of the world.

Among patients with MDR-TB, 7 to 10 percent are extensively drug resistant (XDR-TB) (7), meaning that they are resistant to isoniazid and rifampin and

Tuberculosis

CASE STUDY

A 48-year-old physician-scientist, who had emigrated from China, worked in a microbiology laboratory with TB specimens for several years. Her skin test was negative for TB when she came to the United States, but a blood test was positive after she developed fever, weakness, weight loss, lower chest and abdominal pain, and shortness of breath. She was found to have fluid around her lung (pleurisy). She underwent a pleural biopsy, which grew Mycobacterium tuberculosis. She started taking four medications, and within two months, she had regained her strength and weight. She continued the medicine for even longer than the six months recommended because drug resistance was found. During therapy, she developed joint aches from one of the drugs but finished the course. Despite the drug resistance, the patient recovered and is apparently cured, although she occasionally experiences chest pain when she takes a deep breath.

Comment

In several ways, this patient is a typical vulnerable person. She had increased exposure because of her country of origin and occupation. Her immune system was intact, which may have prevented more serious or fatal disease. The bacteria were resistant to antibiotics, which caused great mental stress to her and her family. She had side effects to the medication, but she ultimately had a good outcome.

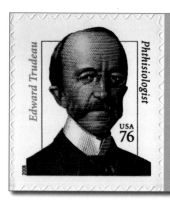

Edward Trudeau

Phthisiologist

USA 76

Dr. Edward Livingston Trudeau was a central figure in the anti-tuberculosis movement. He established the first sanatorium and was founder of the American Sanatorium Association, forerunner of the American Thoracic Society and American Lung Association.

to the next two best classes of medicines (the quinolone family and the inject-able family of antibiotics). The rate of XDR-TB is low in the United States (less than 1 percent), but varies widely around the globe. Precise information on the incidence of XDR-TB is not available for many countries because sensitivity testing for these drugs is not carried out in most of the world.

As drugs are rendered ineffective because of resistance, TB becomes more difficult and expensive to cure. In the United States, the cost of treating a single case of drug-sensitive TB was $8,162 in 2004 (5). In contrast, the average inpa-tient hospital cost for those with MDR-TB who survive the disease was $89,594; the cost rose to $717,555 for those who died (6). The direct costs underestimate the economic burden because they do not include the public health costs of contact screening, tracking, outreach, education, and other expenses—not to mention lost productivity and disruption of the home and workplace.

Although anyone can catch TB, the most vulnerable are those with the greatest exposure. Individuals with decreased immune defense are also at greater risk of developing disease. In addition to HIV, the decreased immunity seen with diabetes, kidney failure, or several medications may tip the balance to favor the tubercle bacilli. There are several, mostly rare, immune defects that also make TB more likely to develop.

If XDR-TB spreads widely, it would pose a colossal public health problem because there would be no good treatment for this easily transmissible infection. XDR-TB has already resulted in quick catastrophic mortality in HIV patients. Rigorous public TB control programs are the cornerstone of efforts to reduce drug resistance (7).

What are we learning about this disease?

Pathophysiology, causes: genetic, environment, microbes

TB is caused by inhaling a few rod-shaped bacteria, *M. tuberculosis*. The bacte-ria, sometimes called tubercle bacilli, must evade the body's defense system, which is formidable in healthy people. A major component of the body's defense is the macrophage, a cell that engulfs and destroys microbes. The bacillus, how-ever, is able to circumvent the macrophage killing and actually multiplies in the macrophage's specialized compartments. Usually, the body wins the battle by suppressing the initial infection, but it may not win the war. Bacilli not destroyed may lie dormant in the cells and tissues (latent TB), but can become active at

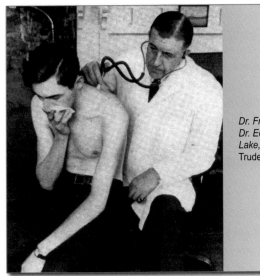

Dr. Francis Berger Trudeau, son of
Dr. Edward Livingston Trudeau, Saranac
Lake, NY, examines a patient. Courtesy:
Trudeau Institute Archives.

any time. Otherwise, healthy persons diagnosed with latent TB have a 5 to 10 percent chance of developing active disease within their lifetime, but persons with HIV and latent TB have a 4.5 percent chance of developing active TB *each year*.

How is it prevented, treated, and managed?

Prevention, treatment, staying healthy, prognosis

Because TB is spread by contact with persons who have it, the first line of TB control is the identification and treatment of active cases. Effective public health programs, however, go beyond this. They identify and treat all known contacts of persons with TB, as well as individuals with latent TB who are at increased risk of developing active disease. The spread of TB occurs primarily through undiagnosed persons, which underscores the importance of tracing individuals who have previously come into contact with an infected person once diagnosis is confirmed.

Patients with active disease are usually isolated until their medications clear their sputum of bacteria. For drug-susceptible cases, this usually occurs within a few days, and isolation within a medical facility is not required. In fact, most patients with TB in the United States are treated as outpatients.

Treatment generally involves taking four drugs under direct medical observation for six months. Side effects are common, but with careful clinical monitoring, they are seldom serious. The outcome is excellent, and cure is complete in most people. Drug-resistant disease is much more difficult to treat, and cure is not assured. Drug resistance develops when patients are treated inadequately. Because a certain number of bacilli are resistant to every drug, taking only one drug kills the sensitive organisms but allows the resistant ones to grow.

Are we making a difference?

Research past, present, and future

The first major breakthrough in controlling the terrible scourge of TB was identifying that it was contagious and caused by bacteria, which led to public health measures. Discovering ways to grow the bacteria in the laboratory, the development of the tuberculin skin test, and x-ray imaging were giant accomplishments of the late 19th and early 20th centuries that allowed accurate diagnoses. A partially effective vaccine, BCG (for Bacille Calmette-Guérin), was developed in the 1920s. In the middle of the 20th century, after decades of research, drugs were discovered that allowed for a permanent cure of TB. The decoding of the entire genomes of humans and *M. tuberculosis* in the 1990s opened new doors of scientific exploration, particularly at the molecular level, and provided new hope that one day TB might be eradicated.

Recent studies have elicited how *M. tuberculosis* becomes dormant when its environment becomes hostile. When the bacteria are in a dormant state, they appear to be resistant to common antituberculous medications. New drug development procedures now test potential agents against both active and dormant forms of the bacilli. Gene array studies are showing that bacterial molecules and molecular pathways can be targets of potential new drugs. Several promising medicines developed this way are now being tested.

As research has uncovered more about the bacteria, the old ways of diagnosing TB are being replaced by newer, faster, and more accurate ones that also give clues to how the human immune system deals with infection. Unraveling the genetic sequence of the bacteria has fostered the development of gene amplification tests that can diagnose the disease and detect drug resistance. These techniques can accomplish in hours or a few days what used to take weeks, thus reducing the chances of a person spreading the disease before being diagnosed and treated.

What we need to cure and eliminate tuberculosis

Even with these advances, progress has been slow, and new breakthroughs are needed to eliminate TB worldwide. Better vaccines must be developed. Fortunately, several are in the early stages of testing. One type of vaccine, similar to most vaccines in use today, could be given to persons who have never had TB to prevent them from getting the disease if they come into contact with it. Another type could enhance natural immunity in persons with latent disease. Yet another form of vaccine could introduce specific biologic molecules into persons with active disease to tip the fight against the organism in favor of the infected person.

Although the current diagnostics are a step forward, better tools still need to be developed. T cells are white blood cells (lymphocytes) that play a central role in the immunity to TB. In the future, the presence and amount of different types of T cells may enable physicians to determine when all the TB bacteria have been killed or, even more beneficially, when someone with latent disease is on the verge of developing active disease and, therefore, should be treated. It could also help determine how long drug-resistant TB needs to be treated.

New drugs also need to be developed to reduce the time it takes to cure a person with TB and to overcome drug resistance. The discovery of the mechanisms of how the bacteria cause disease makes developing drugs of this sort a good prospect. Finding agents that inhibit multiple bacterial metabolic pathways could reduce the length of treatment. For example, killing both active and dormant bacilli could shorten therapy from six months or longer to possibly only a few weeks. Lengthy treatment is a huge hurdle for eliminating the disease.

Advances in the laboratory and new drugs must be tested in the field through clinical trials and then applied in communities through effective public healthcare systems. To eliminate TB in the United States and worldwide, there must be strong leadership to ensure that these advances, along with the experience in dealing with the deadliest epidemic known to man, result in TB control programs in which all nations—rich and poor, with high prevalence and low—can participate.

References

1. Waksman SA. *The Conquest of Tuberculosis.* Berkeley, CA: University of CA Press; 1964.
2. Centers for Disease Control and Prevention (CDC). Trends in tuberculosis—United States, 2008. *MMWR Morb Mortal Wkly Rep* 2009;58:249–253.
3. World Health Organization Web site. Kim JY, Shakow A, Castro A, Vande C, Farmer P. Tuberculosis control. http://www.who.int/trade/distance_learning/gpgh/gpgh3/en/index.html. Accessed January 21, 2010.
4. Dye C, Scheele S, Dolin P, Pathania V, Raviglione MC. Consensus statement. Global burden of tuberculosis: estimated incidence, prevalence, and mortality by country. WHO Global Surveillance and Monitoring Project. *JAMA* 1999;282:677–686.
5. Marks SM. Potential TB treatment cost savings using moxifloxacin-based regimens. *TB Notes* 2006;1:13–15.
6. Rajbhandary SS, Marks SM, Bock NN. Costs of patients hospitalized for multidrug-resistant tuberculosis. *Int J Tuberc Lung Dis* 2004;8:1012–1016.
7. World Health Organization. *Anti-Tuberculosis Drug Resistance in the World. Fourth Global Report.* Geneva, Switzerland: World Health Organization; 2008.

Web sites of interest

CDC Tuberculosis Elimination
www.cdc.gov/tb/

International Standards of Tuberculosis Care
www.thoracic.org/sections/about-ats/assemblies/mtpi/resources/istc-report.pdf

Medline Plus on tuberculosis
www.nlm.nih.gov/medlineplus/**tuberculosis**.html

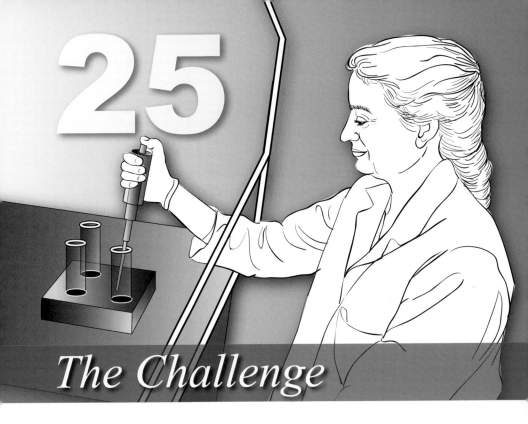

The Challenge

Respiratory disease affects millions of Americans and comes in many forms, common or rare, mild or lethal, acute or chronic, curable or intractable. Regardless of its nature, each lung disease exacts a toll on lives, health, wealth, and happiness. Common to most of these diseases is that they interfere with the ability to breathe, which is terrifying acutely and debilitating chronically. The challenge of curing or eliminating lung diseases is best met through research and application of its findings.

The dawn of the molecular age

The ability today to study complex molecules holds even greater promise than the golden age of bacteriology of the late 1800s. In the second half of the 19th century, the discovery of microbes as a cause of disease marked a revolution in medical science. Methods of isolating, identifying, and culturing bacteria led to an explosion of knowledge. Discovering the cause of these diseases opened the door to further research that explored how these germs thrived and how they could be controlled. Public health measures then reduced or eliminated many diseases. The ability to directly test for an illness led to better diagnoses.

These discoveries brought about the development of antibiotics a half-century later, but even before then, the burden of these diseases greatly declined.

Fortunately, knowledge in science is cumulative. One discovery leads to another and sometimes to dozens more. Breakthroughs may open completely new fields of investigation. Even failed experiments may have great value. The incremental nature of knowledge gained through research makes it an essential element in our hope for developing cures for lung disease in the future.

In today's science, the emphasis is on the precise understanding of what leads to the failure of a molecule, cell, or system. Understanding of the molecular mechanisms is even more significant than was the discovery of disease-causing bacteria in the 19th century. Cellular and molecular systems are far more complicated, but the potential payoffs are vastly greater.

Today, most researchers believe that there is a genetic tendency (possibly due to only a slight fault in the body's chemistry) that renders someone more susceptible to a disease. Coupling this genetic defect with an environmental or chance health risk can lead to a functional breakdown and subsequent illness. Sometimes a series of insults causes disease. Linking genetic abnormalities and environmental stimuli to specific diseases could explain why certain individuals develop a disease and others do not. Among the arguments for this "genes-plus-environment" theory is the fact that identical twins do not always get the same illnesses.

Identification of genetic predispositions alerts individuals with such tendencies to avoid certain environmental factors. For example, an individual with alpha-1 antitrypsin deficiency, which leads to emphysema, is much more likely to suffer dire consequences if exposed to tobacco smoke. An additional benefit of identifying genes predisposing to a certain disease is that the gene products can be studied. Knowing which proteins the gene produces can unravel the underlying mechanism of the disease and help scientists understand the biochemical interactions that lead to it. Replacement or repair of these gene products can lead to new treatments or even cures.

Elements of a cure

It is not too bold to think of each disease as being on a pathway to a cure. Finding a cure is a stepwise process that starts with identifying a problem. Diseases are established by noticing a set of circumstances around one or more health problems. Descriptions of these manifestations, along with an understanding of the clinical setting, help to define the illness. The disease description and associations make up the science of epidemiology, the study of how a disease affects a population.

Progress toward a cure generally does not proceed without understanding the basic mechanisms of the disease—how and where the body's systems have been disrupted. The clearer the understanding of the mechanisms of illness, the more likely that useful diagnostic tests and effective treatments can be found. Understanding the total disease process also allows a more rational approach to prevention and management.

Precisely defining a disease makes research more productive. For example, sepsis, respiratory failure, and chronic obstructive pulmonary disease (COPD) are defined by the clinical presentation and events, not by a precise pathological mechanism. Discovering a single agent for cure of these complex processes is unlikely. Rather, research can help find better ways to manage the diseases, or, potentially, to find a cure for a specific subtype.

On the other hand, a precisely defined disease with a single defect has great potential for a cure because the gene and the molecules it controls can be bypassed or replaced, or the effects of the faulty product can be attenuated. Respiratory distress of the newborn is an example of such a disease. Once the defect—lack of surfactant—was identified, therapy was developed, and the lives of thousands of newborn babies are now being saved every year. Cystic fibrosis and alpha-1 antitrypsin deficiency are other examples of diseases with single-gene defects. Replacement therapy is already available for the latter, though it does not represent a cure.

Identification of a candidate cure or vaccine is only the first step in controlling the disease. Enormous effort, time, and money must be expended to bring promising products through the clinical trials and approval process and eventually to market. Pharmaceutical companies screen between 500 and 10,000 molecules (for both efficacy and toxicity in cells and animals) to find one drug that can be marketed. It is estimated that the cost of bringing a drug to market is greater than $800 million (1). With the great advances in basic science brought on by today's molecular research, the bottleneck in finding a cure is often the clinical trials. The process of recruiting clinical investigators and enrolling a sufficient number of appropriate patients while following the documentation requirements and regulations is difficult and expensive.

Research in the last 20 years has brought great progress in understanding most lung diseases, and some appear close to breakthroughs. With others, however, a cure remains distant, for several possible reasons: The disease could be poorly defined. The cause may be unknown, with a lack of promising leads. There may be limited genetic and mechanistic information, or no animal or adequate marker. Occasionally, previous failed attempts to understand the disease may have discouraged investigators.

Markers

Markers are reliable and readily measured factors that provide a way to monitor disease activity. For example, cholesterol has been closely linked to heart disease. It is much easier to conduct a study of a drug that lowers cholesterol over a few months than to give a drug and follow study subjects for many years in the hope that it will decrease their chance of dying from heart disease. For infectious diseases, the best marker is usually identification of the invading organism itself. When the microbe is too small or too few to be seen or isolated, measuring the body's immune reaction in terms of antibodies often constitutes the necessary marker.

Markers are essential because they allow diagnoses to be easily made and often can be used to grade severity. They are important in leading to a cure because different experimental therapies can be judged by their effects on the marker. Unfortunately, many respiratory diseases do not have good markers. Unlike Papanicolaou (Pap) smears, which test for cervical cancer, sputum examination and x-ray imaging have so far not been trustworthy screening tests for lung cancer.

Applying a cure

Even when a treatment becomes available, it may not be fully utilized. The first effective treatment for tuberculosis was introduced in 1944. The availability of a second drug, para-aminosalicylic acid (PAS), in 1951 allowed a permanent cure in most patients, but 50 years later, the number of cases of tuberculosis in the world was still rising. Although this is largely a problem of healthcare delivery in developing countries, it demonstrates the importance of the healthcare system in aspects of disease management beyond finding a cure.

Difficulties in applying new treatments are several-fold. New drugs have been tested in clinical trials to assure safety and efficacy, but usually in relatively

Lung function with age: nonsmokers, smokers, and those who quit

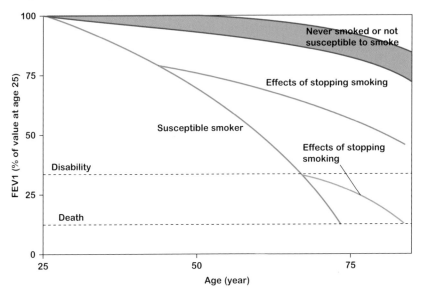

This graph shows the decline in lung function, as measured by forced expiratory volume in one second (FEV1) with age for smokers and nonsmokers. It also shows that quitting smoking can slow the decline in lung function and lead to a longer life. Fletcher C, Peto R. The natural history of chronic airflow obstruction. Br Med J 1977;1:1645–1648.

small numbers of persons in a controlled environment. More experience is usually necessary before the treatment is accepted for patients beyond a clinical trial. Additional experience and study are usually required before the treatment is incorporated into medical guidelines, which are recommendations from experts who have reviewed the evidence for efficacy. Even after new therapies are incorporated into guidelines, their high cost may be a barrier to their use. The emerging field of Comparative Effectiveness Research seeks to distinguish which of competing therapies is better.

What can be done?

Most of these barriers are being addressed. The field of bioinformatics has been developed to analyze the information discerned from complicated systems.

Definition and understanding of diseases have provided a major thrust for research over the last two decades. The pharmaceutical industry has led the way in developing rapid throughput methods to test new compounds, and the search for sound biomarkers is vigorous.

Awareness

An important part of the path to cure is awareness. Millions of people around the globe are unaware of the hazards of smoking and air pollution and the enormous afflictions they cause (2,3). Even in the developed countries, lung disease is often under-recognized and its research is underfunded. The Centers for Disease Control and Prevention in its 2004 monograph, "The Burden of Chronic Diseases and their Risk Factors," listed the top 5 lethal diseases in the United States and discussed all of them except lung disease (4).

Patients, their healthcare providers, and advocacy organizations reach out to the research community and funding agencies to increase awareness for their disease and stimulate research initiatives. Awareness helps identify areas of the greatest need, ensure that promising scientific leads are followed up, and enroll patients in clinical studies.

Awareness is equally important after new therapies become available to teach healthcare providers and the public about their availability and proper use. Imparting new information helps physicians and others prescribe appropriately. It also helps practice preventive behavior and use new treatments safely. For all these reasons, the ATS, along with other international respiratory societies, launched an awareness campaign, declaring 2010 the Year of the Lung.

Research

Research is essential for companies to become leaders in specific areas. New products can advance not only a company but a whole society and can be an engine for extended prosperity. Biomedical research has value to society far beyond products. It can increase employment, build infrastructure, and produce financial gain. Research is the hope for patients suffering from diseases.

It is no accident that the United States is the leader in biomedical research—70 to 80 percent of the total global biomedical research is sponsored by U.S. governmental agencies, U.S.-based foundations, and U.S.-headquartered corporations (2). The United States has benefited most from its research success,

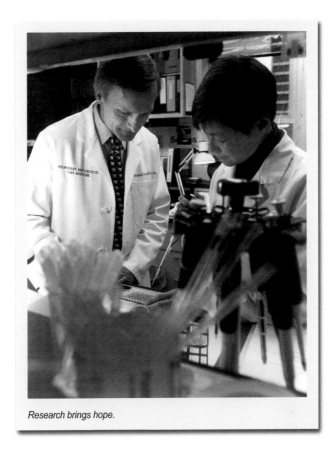

Research brings hope.

but because the benefits of scientific research can be shared by everyone, research gains may be America's greatest gift to the world. Knowledge gained by biomedical research is magnified by sharing. Great advances have come from many nations, and these shared advances have fueled successes in the United States and other countries. Continuation of this rapid pace of acquiring new knowledge requires ongoing international cooperation.

The remarkable success of biomedical research has in part been brought about by the thoughtful planning of the U.S. Congress. Adjusting for inflation, biomedical research funding in the United States grew annually by 7.8 percent from 1994 to 2003, foreshadowing the great advances of today. However, National Institutes of Health and industry funding slowed from 2003 to 2007 and decreased in 2008. Adjusting for inflation, the National Institutes of Health budget decreased by 8.6 percent from 2003 to 2007. Foundations and charities also slowed their funding from 2003 to 2007 compared with a decade earlier (3). For the United States to keep its preeminence in biomedical research, it needs to continue to invest.

Protecting and enhancing breathing throughout the world

Far too many Americans suffer from respiratory disease. The occurrence and importance of asthma, COPD, lung cancer, and sleep apnea are rising, and these and other respiratory conditions affect millions of people. Influenza outbreaks make poignant the vulnerability of our lungs that rely on air shared by almost every living creature. Our dependence on shared air also makes us vulnerable to air pollution, others' cigarette smoke, and, potentially, acts of terrorism.

The answers to the far-ranging question of how to protect and enhance respiratory health require strengthening and enhancing the promising research already under way. Research and application of new knowledge are keys to making even greater gains.

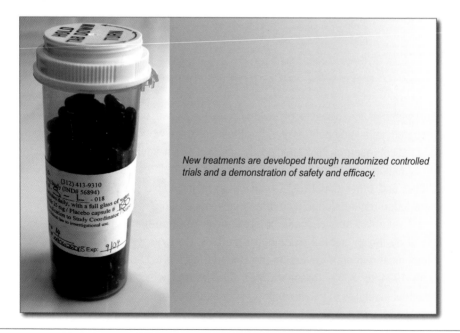

New treatments are developed through randomized controlled trials and a demonstration of safety and efficacy.

Investments in biomedical research have prevented many people from suffering from respiratory diseases. For all, it has brought gains in their length and quality of life. In fact, the consequences of not investing in research are more costly than the dollars spent, especially as the progress made in understanding disease processes is translated into reducing, controlling, curing, and eliminating disease. These advances also help the United States remain an international leader in combating respiratory diseases. This effort provides economic benefits as new discoveries lead to new treatments that open new markets worldwide.

Today, many lung diseases are preventable and treatable, but others still have no effective therapy. Gains have been impressive but the means to make greater gains are even more impressive. Research is giving hope where there was none. The rallying point not only for researchers, clinicians, public health officials, and patients, but for all Americans, should be a cure for all respiratory disease. Society should demand no less.

References

1. DiMasi JA, Hansen RW, Grabowski HG. The price of innovation: new estimates of drug development costs. *J Health Econ* 2003;22:151–185.
2. Global surveillance, prevention and control of chronic respiratory diseases: a comprehensive approach. Bousquet J, Khaltaev N (Editors). World Health Organization 2007.
3. The global burden of disease: 2004 update. World Health Organization 2008.
4. The Burden of Chronic Diseases and their Risk Factors. CDC Department of Health and Human Services 2004.5. Schweitzer SO. *Pharmaceutical Economics and Policy.* 2nd ed. New York, NY: Oxford University Press; 2006.
5. Dorsey ER, de Roulet J, Thompson JP, Reminick JI, Thai A, White-Stellato Z, Beck CA, George BP, Moses H 3rd. Funding of US biomedical research, 2003–2008. *JAMA* 2010;303:137–143.